MOM, DAD...
CAN WE TALK?

HELPING OUR AGING PARENTS WITH THE INSIGHT AND WISDOM OF OTHERS

Written by
Dick Edwards
Mayo Clinic Eldercare Specialist, Retired

And
Mia Corrigan, Jane Danner, Mary Ann Djonne,
Mike Ransom, Angie Swetland

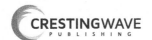
CRESTINGWAVE
PUBLISHING

MOM, DAD... CAN WE TALK?
Helping Our Aging Parents with the Insight and Wisdom of Others

For permission requests, write to the publisher at:
pub@gocwpub.com

ISBN: 978-1-7354135-0-1

A Top Kick imprint from Cresting Wave Publishing, LLC
Published by Cresting Wave Publishing, LLC.

"You buy a book. We plant a tree."

Edited by Christine LePorte and Kris Neely
Cover design: Kris and Laura Neely
Layout design: Lazar Kackarovski

Stock photography: *www.istockphoto.com*

Each of us is someone's child;
many have parents living;
and, all of us should have an older person in our life
to share with, learn from, and care for.

- Dick Edwards

Dedication

To my beloved wife, Pat, and our children, and the hundreds of older persons and their families who have shared their journeys and their wisdoms with us.

Special Thanks

- To Pat Edwards, for fifty-six years of unconditional love, encouragement, and support.
- To Mike Ranson, writer, colleague, and friend, for always being there when needed.
- To Ruth Weispfenning, colleague, and friend, for helping get it all started.
- And to Angie Swetland, Mary Ann Djonne, Mia Corrigan, and Jane Danner for helping make this book better by sharing their personal and professional experiences.

TABLE OF **CONTENTS**

Welcome! As you read, we ask that you stop and think, and remain mindful of the Five 'ates:

evaluate,

anticipate,

communicate,

navigate, and

celebrate your parents' growing older.

PREFACE: WHY A REVISED EDITION?

WELCOME! I'M GLAD YOU found us.

The first edition of *Mom, Dad ... Can We Talk?* was a collaboration with Ruth Weispfenning and Mike Ransom, my friends and colleagues. They provided valuable discipline and inspiration to the process.

By the numbers, the book was a success: it sold more than 7,000 copies. I had the privilege of traveling the country to speak to over 130 audiences of appreciative adult children.

But more gratifying than the numbers is knowing the book and presentations have touched the lives of thousands of families dealing with aging parents' issues and concerns, offering understanding and support, encouragement, insight and perspectives, guidance, and lessons learned from the experiences of others.

So, why a revised edition of *Mom, Dad ... Can We Talk?*

There are three good reasons:

First, the topic of adult children and aging parents is both timeless and timely. More people are living longer, numerically and proportionally. Consequently, more families than ever before are engaged in some level of eldercare. Adult children are challenged to balance the stresses and strains of work, parenting, and family life with aging parents' changing needs. It can be a lot to deal with.

Second, my meetings with groups of adult children gave rise to the need to address additional topics not included in the first edition. In this revised edition, I am joined by Guest Contributors who have the personal and professional experience needed to address important new topics:

○ In the section titled *Encore,* Angie Swetland looks at how grandchildren can be helped to understand the aging process and maintain their unique relationship with their aging grandparents.

○ Mary Ann Djonne teams with Mia Corrigan to help families with the unique concerns of aging parents who have a special needs adult child.

○ Jane Danner talks about how the sudden intrusion of external reality, like a pandemic, complicates and brings even more significant challenges in our care for aging parents.

Finally, it's the recognition that *Mom, Dad ... Can We Talk?* is well suited for aging parents to read and discuss alongside their concerned adult children. The book also serves as an icebreaker for families, particularly those who have discomfort having the conversations that will be so helpful in the end. Lastly, it gives both sides—aging parents and adult children—a framework, a guide from which to begin. "Let's read and discuss it."

I often hear aging parents declare emphatically: "I don't want to be a burden on my kids." I've said it myself. Have you? When you think about it, aging parents are burdens to the extent that we don't plan, don't anticipate our needs and preferences, and communicate to our kids what they need to know for "when the time comes." It's one more thing we do for our kids.

Mom, Dad ... Can We Talk? lends itself to group discussion in adult learning classes, book clubs, and family gatherings. Adult children are eager to share their stories about dealing with aging parents and to learn from others' experiences. Included in this revised edition is a flexible, easy-to-use guide for group discussion.

So please, read on. And along the way, stop. Think. And have conversations.

I am sure you will find insights and perspectives to help ensure success as your parents age.

Dick Edwards

INTRODUCTION:
SETTING THE STAGE

"Each of us is someone's child; many have parents living, and all of us should have an older person in our life to share with, learn from, and care for."

Dick Edwards

URING MY THIRTY-FIVE-YEAR CAREER in older adult services, I was privileged to share in the lives of hundreds of older people. I formed supportive relationships with them and their families. I was called upon daily to offer support and counsel.

As I reflect on my experiences, I have concluded that adult children generally have good intentions. Still, they are often ill-prepared to make the best of relationships with their parents, manage the myriad issues common to the later years in family life, and maximize the opportunities for good times.

Over and over, I heard adult children say, "I feel a responsibility for my parents. I care. I want to do the right thing. What is the right thing? I welcome help."

Mom, Dad...Can We Talk? is my response to their pleas. It draws from my years of working with older people. It shares insights about how adult children and their families can manage the challenges and get the most out of their parents' final years. I share many personal stories, including lessons from a survey I conducted of one hundred adult children who are on—or who have recently completed—the journey with their older parents.[1]

---

1 Numerous quotes from those responding to the survey appear in callout boxes throughout the book.

The Pew Research Center estimates that 77 million baby boomers are simultaneously dealing with their life issues, their children's needs, and the needs of an elderly parent or parents.

I've written this book for them.

For some families, this stage of life—when parents grow old—is a walk in the park. Relationships are tidy, everyone communicates, resources are available, choices are sufficient, decisions come easy, and the later years are golden.

For other families, perhaps most, these years are characterized by the fear of the unknown: fear of what's to happen, of failure, of not doing the right thing. It's also a time of frustration with parents, siblings, and "the system." It's a draining push-pull that taps and saps time, energy, and resources.

People ask: Who does better at this stage of family life when adult children face the challenges of aging parents? From my experience, families who seem to do better share four things in common.

First, they enter this stage with a proper attitude, preferably a positive attitude. A positive attitude usually carries the day and helps ensure success.

Second, they enter with some basic understanding of the aging process and solid working knowledge of their family dynamics. Who in the family can play a role in caring for aging parents? What are their strengths?

Third, families do better if they have realistic expectations of themselves, their parents, their family members, friends, and the community resources intended to help.

And, finally, families who "plan ahead" clearly seem to do better. Yes, success in this stage of family life can be planned; families who evaluate, anticipate, and communicate tend to succeed.

There are many references, guides, and compendiums available that assist adult children in helping their aging parents. Much of this information resides on the Internet. Google the phrases "living will," "healthcare directive," or "nursing homes in Minnesota," for example, and you'll see long lists of sources that provide information about the topics.

However, some information, the personal and practical things you need to know, isn't easily found.

This book addresses these situations. It's foundational, fundamental.

Mom, Dad...Can We Talk? looks at roles and relationships among family members. It acknowledges and respects family history to help gauge present-day expectations. It identifies areas of potential difficulty as well as areas of possible pleasure.

It asks you to stop and think, anticipate, and start conversations with your parents and those who care about them. And it also deals with a fundamental distinction: growing old versus aging.

In this book, we talk about the importance of gaining perspectives and insight. We seek to help our parents grow older and age because how we come to view aging and how we understand aging is fundamental. In many ways, how we view and appreciate our parents' aging will affect our behavior towards them as they age.

Consider, then: Growing older really is a vastly different experience than aging.

Over the life span, growing older has obvious perks and pleasures. For example, when we get older, we can sit at the big people's table for family gatherings, get a two-wheeled bike, and obtain a driver's license. We can graduate from high school, leave our parents' home, launch our adult life, start a career, get a place of our own, and maybe get married and raise a family. When we get older, we can retire from work and enjoy life!

These are some perks and pleasures of growing older.

But, aging, not so much.

No amount of nips or tucks, replacement parts, lotions, or potions will prevent the dynamic, unstoppable aging process. Aging is biological, physiological, and anatomical. It's functional, and it's cognitive. Net-net: aging is inevitable. And it can be unpleasant.

Understand, too, that the universal hallmark of aging is loss. As we age, we can lose hearing, vision, even taste, smell, and touch. Our general health can decline. We can lose physical strength, gait, energy, and stamina. We can lose status and self-esteem, treasured relationships, options, independence, and control.

So, when your parents resist the idea of moving, or dad fights you on giving up his driver's license, or mother her checkbook, consider all their losses. And the natural desire not to lose anything more.

Aging is loss, and no one likes to lose.

Imagine what aging is like for your parents. We can't really empathize because we don't know. We've never been old.

Let our parents tell us.

Sympathize, seek to understand, respect what it means to them, and gauge your expectations accordingly.

Also, understand what your parents' aging means to you. Are you OK with the reality of their aging? How is it for other family members? Your sister or your brother? Your children? You might be surprised.

How we feel about our parents' aging will influence our behaviors towards them as they age.

———————————

I asked my colleagues Ruth Weispfenning and Mike Ransom to help me write this book. Ruth is a licensed social worker and director of resident services at the retirement community where I served as administrator. She is a talented problem-solving coach. Time and again, I watched Ruth calmly guide families through stress-filled situations.

Mike is a memoirist who has written over a dozen books. He has the gift of asking questions, listening, gently probing, and translating what he discerns into the written word. Mike has a particular fondness for older people. He delights in helping them tell their life stories for family and friends to treasure.

We tried to make *Mom, Dad...Can We Talk?* an enjoyable read about topics common to a critical stage in family life, one often challenging to manage. We invite you to reflect on the stories and insights we share, but most importantly, to find things to draw from them as you share this time with your parents and with older persons in your life.

It's worth it.

CHAPTER 1

CURTAIN UP ON **ACT 3!**

"What is difficult as an adult child is not knowing what the future holds for my parents. What might happen next that we will need to face together? I fear the phone's ringing. I feel like I'm living on the edge of something dreadful."

IMAGINE YOU AND YOUR family are starring in a three-act play. Act 1 features your growing up years. It's a fun time, safe and predictable. Your parents are central to your universe. Siblings and friends, relatives and neighbors, teachers and coaches round out the cast. You are learning, growing, and becoming. Family roles and relationships are formed, and private and family foundations are laid.

Act 2 spotlights your young adult years; you are consumed with completing your education, starting a family, and embarking on a career. Siblings move from the parental nest and see each other less often: on holidays, weddings, baptisms, and funerals. While not incidental to your hectic life, your parents participate, but they are on their own and rarely share center stage.

Before you know it, the curtain lifts on Act 3. You've become middle-aged. The cast of characters has changed. Some have gone; others have joined. At the start of this act, you look over your shoulder and say, "Who's that over there? Oh my God, it's my parents. Where have they been? They can't be in their eighties, can they? Have I been that self-engrossed? What have I missed?"

The close-knit family in Act 1 that drifted apart somewhat in Act 2 must now regroup in Act 3 to grow older with their parents. Success in your family's Act 3 boils down to how well you and your family anticipate needs, educate yourselves, communicate, delegate, navigate issues and opportunities, and learn to celebrate the simple things in life with your parents.

Some families do these things well, while others must work harder. We presume the curtain is up on Act 3 of your family play for this book's purposes.

> Those last years were challenging at times. But we took them head-on. My, what joys we shared.

Yes, for many families, this act can be a glorious climax to lives well lived. But for others, this time may be a regrettable close...to what could have been. We've written this book to help you achieve the former.

One way to help avoid that "what could have been" scenario is to remember this: children, young and old, learn by example. Your children are watching you, taking mental notes as they see you interact with your aging parents.

Remember this as well: what they observe, hear, feel, and experience will help set the stage when you are the aging parent in Act 3.

CHAPTER 2

GROWING OLDER
HAPPENS

"I noticed that when my parents stopped trying to stay young,
they began to enjoy growing older."

MANY OF OUR PARENTS enjoy active, independent lives. However, all of us must sooner or later come to grips with the reality that our parents are growing older. In doing so, they may well experience the loss of loved ones, health, stamina, and even independence. And they too realize that ultimately, they will die.

As we do with most troubling thoughts in life, we push them into the far corner of our minds.

Though the aging process itself has not changed much across human history, what has changed is that, on average, humanity lives longer every year. The current life expectancy for adults in the United States is 79.9 years, which means your parents have a 50% chance of living into their eighties and beyond.

Therefore, each year more of us in the "sandwich generation" (those sandwiched between caring for our aging parents and supporting our own children) will not only be living longer—we'll be doing so with parents who are in their eighties and nineties!

Don't fear the process of your parents growing older. And don't lament it. Those denied the privilege of older parents—through illness or accident—would gladly trade places with you.

Your growing-older parents are a gift. Celebrate them!

That said, we are not soft-pedaling the fact that growing older can be difficult. Our friend Lois, summing up all her eighty-nine years, said: "We're all trying to endure the indignities of aging as gracefully as we can."

Our challenge is to help our parents do this gracefully and with dignity.

The media can paint a gloomy picture of growing old by playing on our nursing home fears. A TV ad shows a young daughter sitting and holding hands with her dad on his porch's front steps. The ad touts a new medication for treating mild forms of dementia. The daughter says, "I was so afraid I would have to put Dad in a nursing home." Sweet, but let's face reality. If her father needs to be in a nursing home, he needs to be in a nursing home. It is doubtful that a single pill will prevent that.

Another slice of reality: nursing homes and similar facilities are, in a significant number of cases, changing and adapting to the realities of today's aging parents. The key is education about the state of such facilities.

When a family begins dealing with an aging parent, typically, they only know two extremes:

○ care at home
○ spending the rest of their days in a "nursing home"

Today, there are many options in between, and, as we said, this industry is transforming rapidly. As evidenced by the continued lengthening of the human life span we mentioned earlier, these facilities have a changing role in the continuum of life care and services.

> From now on, if older people enter a nursing home, it may well be at a later age—and for a shorter stay.
>
> As Mom slowed down, we set our sights on the level of activity we thought she could handle.
>
> It was enough to help keep her engaged.

Most of us don't sit around the dinner table with our parents and talk about aging and dying. Death is often a taboo family topic saved for the bedside as a parent takes his or her last breath. In the author's experience, we've learned that seniors are more comfortable with the topic than one might expect.

Here's just one example. Seniors are often asked if they have written end-of-life wishes:

- ○ Do they wish to be resuscitated?
- ○ Do they wish to be intubated?
- ○ Which family members should be contacted?
- ○ Which funeral home do they prefer?

While these may seem like awkward questions to ask, many seniors will respond, "Oh, we've already contacted the funeral home, and everything is taken care of."

Our experience shows you'd probably be surprised at how much thinking your parents have done about their dying. And to be candid, you may discover they are more accepting of it than you are. It's just that they haven't shared many of their thoughts about it with you. After all, it's not a popular dinner table conversation topic.

Take the lead from your parents and don't feel timid about the topic of their dying.

Now that we've reminded you of the obvious—that everyone dies and that growing older can be fraught with difficulties—let's put those thoughts aside. Death and despair are, after all, not this book's central themes. Since we've just established how it ends, we want to help you make the most of your time with your parents.

Our focus is on life and family relationships.

Yes, it is rough getting older. Many people smooth their path by reaching back into their experience to apply the coping skills and "situation handling" experiences life has presented. With this, they make the best of growing older. It's a good start.

To be sure, some people are naturally better than others at doing this. Some have always been able to roll with the punches better than others. People who have a history of coping with adversity and toughing things out might view aging as just another challenge. "I've marched up to this sort of thing before," they'll say, "and I'm sure I'll do quite nicely, thank you."

We've learned that nearly everyone experiences aging just differently enough that we need to respect each variation. Aging provides chances for people to shine. Some seniors come alive in their twilight years and show a new or different side. As evidenced in the following story, kids are surprised to see what Mom can do on her own now that Dad is gone.

An adult daughter worried that her mother would curl in a corner and crumble after her husband died.

Instead, she was soon planning a cruise to the Caribbean.

The daughter reported to her friends, "Mother just called to ask if I could stop by her apartment to help her choose which bathing suit to take on her upcoming cruise.

"And she surprised me even more by asking, 'Oh, by the way, would you be willing to join me?'"

The authors have seen many families share the ups and downs of aging, all while experiencing their way through their parents' later years. There will be challenges; life always makes sure of that. But the times can be enriching and fun.

One of their joys, while growing older, was watching their children become wholesome, productive adults.

Families, realizing that they don't have an unlimited amount of time left with Mom and Dad, often deal with issues that have been on the table for years.

They bury hatchets.

In one family, the mother and daughter—who had not spoken for twenty years—restarted their relationship through a brief visit while the mother was in a nursing home. Neither could even remember why they had stopped talking to each other.

They find closure over a critical issue in their past in other families, such as never telling nieces and nephews that their mother had been married once before.

In still other families, parents and children are no longer shy about saying "I love you" when they meet or depart.

And significantly, at some point in their lives, many adult children realize that regardless of how well they like their mother or father, they should also respect them. The teachings and writings of the world's faiths nearly all speak of the important role of the elderly in the family.

Finally, since death comes to all of humanity, one must keep living until it does, as Sophie believes in the following story.

> Sophie was a delightful lady with a loving husband. She had terminal breast cancer and had come to the nursing home to die.
>
> Her condition stabilized shortly after she came in, so she began planning a vacation. The nursing staff asked the administrator to talk with Sophie about the denial of her illness.
>
> As he began a discussion with Sophie, she said, "I know I am dying, but I plan to live until I die."
>
> Sophie didn't live long enough to take that vacation.
>
> But she provided a powerful lesson on living with a positive attitude.

So, the authors' advice at this point is simple: put this book down and call your parents. Just because.

CHAPTER 3

SEEK FIRST TO
UNDERSTAND

*"The older I become, the better I understand
what my mother's going through."*

ADULT CHILDREN NEED TO pause a moment in their rush-here-rush-there lives to put themselves in their parents' shoes. As with many situations, one key to helping a parent grow older is to seek first to understand. In this, empathy is vital.

Genuinely try to imagine what it's like for your parent. Try your best to see the world through his or her eyes. Educate yourself about the entire situation so you can correctly gauge expectations and find your role. Try for a moment to imagine what it would be like to be eighty-five. Imagine you had to experience and live with:

- a cataract in your right eye
- arthritis in both hands and both feet
- a hearing aid in your left ear
- corns on both feet
- a bladder you can't trust
- and a knee that really does need replacement

That's your physical situation all day, every day.

What about your mental and emotional condition? Imagine the emotional hammer blows of having siblings, lifelong friends, business associates, neighbors, and maybe a spouse or even one of your children die, one by one, as you live on?

How would you feel if you could no longer drive? Or if you fell in the shower and could not help yourself up?

> As their health failed, I began to feel more like a parent to my parents.
>
> And I realized the roles were reversing.

But you don't have to pretend to be eighty-five. One day you may well be. And then you'll probably discover that your eighty-five is as unique and different as you are from your parents. And their eight-five years.

How you experience and manage age is shaped by years of behavior, your acquired and natural coping skills, your expectations, and the randomness of your unique genetic makeup. For some people, it's a snap. For other people, it's a grueling, uphill climb.

So, as any eighty-five-year-old can tell you: it's best not to generalize about age. It's better to educate yourself.

> When Phil's eighty-year-old father laments, "It's tough getting older,"
>
> Phil tries never to respond, "I know how you feel."
>
> Phil has experienced many things in his life. Still, he has no idea what waking up one morning in an eighty-year-old body feels like, either physically or emotionally.
>
> Phil also has no idea what emotions are triggered when his father realizes that he has a finite number of times remaining to enjoy what means most to him.
>
> "My gosh, this could be my last Thanksgiving with my family."
>
> Or,
>
> "Spring is my favorite time of year. How many more will I be able to enjoy in this house?"

When a parent says, "It's tough getting older," you have an opportunity. To learn!

Say something like, "Can I please know more about what you're referring to specifically? I have no real frame of reference, but maybe I could learn something from what you're going through."

Then...listen.

Quietly and compassionately.

Hear what they say—and try to understand what they mean.

And this is important: they aren't necessarily looking for you to solve their problems or even to relate literally to those problems one-on-one.

They may simply want someone with whom to share their thoughts. They may hope just to be heard out, to know someone cares enough to listen.

Please don't rush to try to make growing older what you think might be easier for them. Or to try and change it into something it's not. Your dad may not be the same as you remember him. The key is to understand where he's at today.

Empathizing with your parents builds a good foundation for the insights we will share in the remainder of this book. Your parents will be more receptive to your involvement in their growing-older process when they see that you're really and actively listening—and trying to see things from their perspective.

But remember what we've just learned: you really don't know much about what they're going through. So, listen more, talk less, and take care about giving too much advice too soon.

CHAPTER 4

SOME THINGS
NEVER CHANGE

"I know this is true: Parents never stop being parents.
While circumstances may have changed and roles may have reversed,
I'm still the child and must let Dad be the parent.
It's what I'll want, too."

YOUR PARENTS WERE A couple. Then they had a child or children, and the couple's "identification" moved to "a family." That's what they've always known: a couple plus a kid(s) equals a family. Also, the joys they knew as a couple grew with the evolution of "family."

As the children in this example, we started our life surrounded by this family and the joys of a family from a child's perspective. To us, a family was always a child or children plus parents. That's what we've always known.

If we are lucky, we'll also end our life surrounded by the joys of family. Whatever happens to us between our birth into the family and our passing away from it lies the groundwork for who we become.

Our "in-between" time might include going away to college or joining the military, perhaps. We might marry, move to another town, start our first "real" job, and start our own family. Also, in this in-between time, the physical relationships with our family typically change as well. How far we live from home, how often we visit our parents, and how often we see our siblings contribute to the family's ever-evolving dynamic.

But the dynamic, engrained, from-birth emotional and familial relationships within our family typically don't change drastically.

At the beginning of this book, we likened our years with our family to a three-act play.

Let's say Act 1 covers your childhood years at home. The audience sees that Mom is goodhearted but has a dominant personality. They see Dad as a hard-working but passive gentleman. They see sister Sarah as the kindest person on planet Earth, but they also see brother Larry as just a total jerk. And—they see that Mom and Dad like Sarah the best. She can do no wrong in their eyes.

Act 2 covers the speeding chronicle of your young adult years.

Before we know it, the curtain rises on Act 3. In this act, the audience sees an older version of the cast from Acts 1 and 2.

Mom is still a dominant-but-goodhearted mom. Dad takes his work a bit easier than before, but he's still just as passive. Larry is still a jerk. And Sarah is still outstanding, impossibly precious, and still the "chosen" child.

> I think, being the oldest child, I was looked upon to take care of things.

Life kind of just works that way.

As such, it's probably wise for you to acknowledge that relationships exhibited in Act 1 of your family play—like them or not—will probably be there in Act 3. While we like to believe we can change, there is truth in the adage, "Some things never change."

The authors are time and again baffled when we see families ignoring the fact that some things really do never change. For example:

○ Why should a brother expect things and behaviors from his sister even though the sister has never shown competence—or even interest—in doing such a thing or exhibiting such behavior?

○ A son who has always been chronically short of money may not be the best person to hold Dad's power of attorney.

○ Why should a daughter whose house is a cluttered mess be entrusted to organize Mom's move to assisted living? She can't do so.

In short, why, now, in their parents' later years, would families expect members to shine in an area they never excelled in before?

Each of us begins Act 3 of our family drama with our family history's good and bad baggage. We must deal with that baggage because we need to acknowledge our family for who we are and build a foundation for dealing with our aging parents' issues and opportunities.

The following conversation among four adult children, each a successful businessperson, shows their reluctance to tell Mom it's time for her to move from independent to assisted living. Though they love their mom, they know she doesn't like to hear unpleasant news.

"You tell her," says one.

"No, you tell her," adds the second.

"I'm not telling her," declares the third.

"Don't look at me," pleads the fourth.

These are not four little boys arguing about who should tell their mom that they just broke the garage window. These are four grown men, each successful in adult life and titans of business. Yet, when it comes time to tell their mother she must move from her independent living apartment to an assisted living setting because she needs reminders about her medications and assistance getting dressed, they lose a good deal of their steely resolve...

They vigorously debate who should break the news.

"You're the oldest. It should come from you. She's always respected your opinion over ours."

"Are you crazy? The last thing I'm going to do is walk into her apartment and tell her we're moving her out. She still tells me to keep my elbows off the table and to chew with my mouth closed."

As a general statement, parents tend to value the opinion of their eldest child. In the following story told by an adult child from a family of six children, Einar, rather than Eleanor, will be consulted for his opinion, simply because he's the oldest.

Growing up, we were a close-knit family—three brothers, three sisters, mom, and dad. We were a farm family of the classic Norwegian Lutheran tradition. Everyone worked hard and contributed to family life. Einar was the oldest. Mother thought he could do no wrong. Sometimes we wondered if he could do anything right. (Just kidding, Einar.)

Brother Einar took over the family farm and worked alongside Dad. As adults, we remained close-knit, returning to the family farm often and gladly for holidays and any occasion we could deem special. Mother was the spirit, the glue.

After Dad died and Mother's health began to fail, she became the primary focus of family concern. She had complicated health issues. Our single sister, Eleanor, had a profession related to caring for older people, so she became the family equivalent of 911 when it came to Mother and her needs. Eleanor did everything.

For months and months, Eleanor monitored Mother's situation, coordinated and orchestrated. She talked with the doctors, the social workers, and the array of healthcare professionals trying to help our mother. Eleanor researched the options, reviewed them all with Mother, and communicated thoroughly and faithfully with the rest of us. She was the go-to person who helped us understand and do the right thing. We did what Eleanor asked.

Everyone greatly appreciated Eleanor. She and Mother grew closer. Eleanor made certain Mother maintained her dignity and her pivotal role in the family. Mother still ran things from her room in the nursing home and still presided at family gatherings on the farm.

When Eleanor and Mother met with the surgeons to discuss leg amputation because of complications from diabetes, Mother listened carefully, thoughtfully reviewing each option and its consequences.

With the ever-faithful Eleanor at her side, the doctor assured Mother that it would have to be her decision. Rather than turning to Eleanor, Mother turned to the surgeon and said, "I'll have to see what Einar has to say. He's the eldest, you know."

No discussion about family dynamics surrounding concerns and care for an aging parent would be complete without mentioning the "out-of-town" sibling. Let's next hear from Keith, an adult child who lives far from his parents.

> For years, my sister and her family enjoyed the benefits of proximity and ease of access to our parents. She and they lived in the same city. Mother and Dad attended all the grandchildren's school and church programs, Little League games, music recitals, birthday gatherings, prom nights, and graduations.
>
> They were tightly woven into the daily fabric of my sister's family life. I was envious.
>
> I lived 210 miles away with my family. Our trips home were infrequent and generally associated with holiday celebrations or family funerals.
>
> As our parents grew older and their needs for support and care increased, my sister, the sibling living closest, became the twenty-four/seven caregiving daughter. I, the out-of-town sibling, was no longer envious.

So how should the out-of-town sibling participate in his or her parents' Act 3?

Some siblings adopt a "blow in, off, and out" approach on the less-than-useful side. They typically make a big deal out of coming to visit Mom or Dad (blow in). Then, they express all sorts of "helpful" suggestions to you, the sibling who lives in the same town with Mom or Dad (blow-off). And finally, they catch the next stagecoach out of Dodge (blow-out).

While that behavior is less than useful, it also creates a false impression of, say, Mom's real state. When the out-of-town sibling is in town, Mom's on center stage. She's on an energy high. She's dressed in her best and looks great.

However, the reality is different as you, the down-the-street-from-Mom sibling, knows, "This is NOT the mom that I deal with every day!"

So, what do we suggest to the out-of-town sibling?

First, please remember that Mom may be putting on a show just for you. Whether you realize it or not, being with the family for a day is much different from being with them every day. In this example, Mom has put her issues on hold until you leave.

Next, as the out-of-town sibling, you should regularly express gratitude to your other siblings who care for their parents day-to-day:

○ Maybe a note that says, "Thanks, I appreciate all you're doing for the folks—I know it isn't easy."

○ Perhaps some unexpected flowers delivered to their door.

○ Possibly an offer to give respite by coming to town for a few days to look after the parent(s) so the in-town sibling can go away and get some rest and recreation.

Whatever the form of expressed gratitude, it's vital that you—the out-of-town sibling— acknowledge your in-town sibling's heavy load and that you appreciate their efforts.

Family dynamics play critical roles when the time comes to help parents grow older and navigate their Act 3. Identify and consider your family dynamics and learn to work within their constraints, realities, and boundaries.

Understand these relationships are there, they have been the way they are for a long time, and you must accept them at face value and as they are and not as you might wish them to be. And try hard NOT to take things personally.

Across the scope and scale of your parents' Act 1, 2, and 3, family history helps explain the present as much as it helps gauge expectations going forward.

CHAPTER 5

CARING
CONVERSATIONS

"The conversations didn't come easy. I thought it was Mom's
reluctance until I realized it was mine."

G ENERALLY, REGARDLESS OF OUR age, we desire to please our
parents. We want to do the right things for them to the extent our
physical and financial capabilities allow.

To do the right things, as they and we grow older, we need to exchange
information with them.[2]

Some information to be shared is practical and factual:

O   Where do your parents do their banking?

O   Who is their broker, lawyer, doctor?

O   Do they have a will?

O   Do they have a burial plot?

O   Where do they keep the key to their safe deposit box?

Other information is quite personal and emotional:

O   What would Mom like her family to do should she develop
dementia?

O   When it's time, what kind of funeral arrangements would Dad
like?

---

2   Wouldn't it be helpful if your parents authored a definitive reference manual entitled, *What to Do
If I Get Daffy, Difficult, or Die,* and handed it to you in Act 3 of your family play? Yes; that would
be nice!

In addition to the information you would like from your parents, there are facts and feelings you want to share with them. A practical fact could be, "Here's how you can reach me in an emergency when I'm traveling overseas on business."

The personal feeling might be, "How will I ever repay you for all the grief I caused you during my college years?"

In the absence of the "What to Do If..." reference manual, you need to have a conversation(s) with your parents. In a conversation, remember to ask, listen, and then, if necessary, talk.

These conversations become the foundation of your remaining time with your parents, and they ofttimes go something like this:

- ○ "Mom, Dad, there are things you need to tell me, things I need to know."
- ○ Or, "Mom, Dad, there are things I need to tell you, things I need you to know."

The authors refer to these as "The Caring Conversations."

In them, facts and feelings are exchanged, parent-to-child, and child-to-parent. Caring conversations help remove the guesswork surrounding what you and your parents need, think, and feel. They establish a foundation and give direction to meeting their needs. And often, yours.

We all find ourselves failing to have essential conversations with those we care most about throughout a lifetime. Sometimes we remonstrate with ourselves because:

- ○ We don't say what needs to be said
- ○ We don't talk about what we feel in our hearts
- ○ We often can't find words or muster the courage to express these thoughts
- ○ Maybe we feel these talks invade our parents' privacy or acknowledge their mortality

We've seen that caring conversations often occur within the context of naturally occurring opportunities—if you are mindful of being awake in and at the moment.

For example, a naturally occurring opportunity might follow a parent's visit to a friend in the hospital, as Sharon discovered in the following situation:

After seeing her best friend of forty years in a hospital bed after a debilitating stroke and awaiting transfer to a nursing home, Sharon's mother said: "Boy, I sure wouldn't want to live like that."

Sharon seized the moment. "Really? Let's talk about that. What would you want to have done?"

Another naturally occurring opportunity might come when a parent voices concerns about a friend's health. Martin tells of beginning a caring conversation with his father after hearing him comment about his golf partner Lawrence:

Martin's dad expressed concern for Lawrence. "He drives like crazy, some days he smells, and some days he totally forgets our tee time.

"His kids should do something; they should show more interest."

It was a perfect opening for Martin: "Dad, what would you want us kids to do if those times ever come with you?"

The subject of when your parents' health indicates they should no longer live at home is always a difficult conversation. Suppose your parents have a friend who has had to deal with such a situation. In that case, it's a perfect, naturally occurring opportunity to discuss the topic. In the following story, an adult child tells about a caring conversation that he and his brother had with their parents after seeing two of the parents' friends undergo a stressful situation:

Clarence and Lucille were our parents' best friends.

Lucille had debilitating health issues that kept her in a wheelchair. Clarence, a gentle, nurturing soul, cared for Lucille twenty-four/seven for many years.

His devotion took its toll.

When their only child, Nancy, suggested putting Lucille in a nursing home, Clarence became angry with her and felt devastated.

Over the years, they had never talked about what would happen "if."

When my brother and I ultimately talked with our parents about Clarence and Lucille's situation, we finally did talk about their "what if."

It was a caring conversation.

A caring conversation need not occur in a tense or difficult setting. Some talks and some topics seem safer while doing basic things around the house like:

- Washing dishes after a family dinner
- Enjoying a sit-down and a cup of coffee
- Snapping beans in the garden
- Tending to everyday chores

Adult children often have meaningful conversations with their parents while riding in the car—especially at night. Maybe it's the soothing hum of the engine. Perhaps it's that people keep their eyes on the road, thus avoiding eye contact. It could be the comforting blanket of darkness. Or maybe it's that while driving, you keep moving ahead, and things are left behind. Whatever the reason, people do seem to open up.

Know that timing is everything—and that when you know a conversation must be had, you seize the moment.

The following story tells how Andy began a caring conversation with his mother, Marge, on the ride home from a family member's funeral:

Marge and Andy drove the forty miles home after Uncle Norbert's funeral. Norbert was Marge's youngest brother and her last living sibling. Norbert had two sons, one daughter, and six grandchildren. His wife, Grace, died several years ago.

The funeral was traditional, with visitation the night before, an open casket, and a little lunch in the church basement afterward.

As they drove, Andy asked his mother, "So, what did you think of the service?"

At first, Marge was tentative. But with some encouragement, a few miles behind them, and some open-ended questions, she began to talk.

Before long, she began to speak about things she would like for her service in a soft voice. She suggested some readings and songs, a few remarks from the grandchildren, and the service's spirit—a spirit of celebration.

Andy didn't make any judgments and didn't offer any commentary.

Instead, he listened and made mental notes. He used this shared experience, his uncle Norbert's funeral, to grow his understanding of what would please his mother and what she would want when the time came.

After a comfortable silence, Andy did ask his mother if she thought they should write this information down for future reference. She replied without hesitation,

"Well, I suppose so, but I'm not going yet!" She promised Andy she would tell him if she changed her mind on any of the specifics.

Deal.

What a pleasant, memorable ride home.

As you have a caring conversation, keep in mind something we mentioned a few pages back: parents never stop being parents. Though circumstances and roles may have changed and even reversed, you are still their child to them.

So do your best to let Mom and Dad parent you. When you think about this, we are sure you'll agree it is what you will want someday, too.

Another essential key to effective, caring conversations is not to underestimate the power of a simple thank-you.

For example, on Veterans Day one year, Gilbert took the time to say to his octogenarian father, "Thanks, Dad, for the time you served in World War II. I know you sacrificed a lot, and I've always appreciated it."

Like many a crusty war veteran, Gilbert's dad said little. He shrugged his shoulders as if to say, "Oh, it was nothing." He's from a generation that, as a rule, doesn't express feelings like Gilbert's generation. But that doesn't mean his emotions don't run as deep.

I could never express my love for Mom and Dad in my own words, so I let Hallmark say it for me.

After Mom died, I found a box containing nearly every card I sent her.

I was glad they meant a lot to her.

A key word of warning seems appropriate here. Many folks just wait too long to have caring conversations with their parents. That's a shame for a variety of reasons, as you can no doubt imagine. But it's also a shame because when this overdue conversation does occur, it is almost a guarantee that the outcome will be less than optimal.

Avoid that. Be mindful of opportunities. Anticipate—then communicate.

As was mentioned briefly before, your parents' Act 3 can also be a perfect time to bury old family or relationship hatchets. Experience has shown us that doing so will usually occur in a caring conversation that begins:

○ "You know, Dad, I've always wanted to tell you how sorry I was for..."

○ Or, "Mom, I've never been able to say this until now, but did you know..."

That said, here's an example of a family who sadly couldn't find a way to bury the hatchet:

Donald and Doris were a wonderful couple, well into their eighties, who had one child, Bill. For reasons unknown to anyone outside these three, the parents and son had not spoken or even seen each other for three decades.

Donald was eventually transferred to a local nursing home. And when Doris died, Bill came to see his dad.

The trust officer asked Donald if he could take Bill to visit his parents' house so he could see where his parents had spent the past thirty years.

Donald gave his approval.

As the son and trust officer entered the house, the son immediately saw numerous childhood pictures of himself on the shelves and walls.

The trust officer said, "You were always a big part of their lives."

Overwhelmed, Bill wept.

The authors have also heard one version or another of the following story from scores of people:

I took comfort in the hospice nurse telling me that hearing was the last sense to be lost in dying.

I spoke the words I needed to say.

But I wish I had said them earlier to hear her response.

We have been present at many hospital and hospice settings where a parent's death is imminent. Family has gathered. The parent is unresponsive. Hands are wringing. A fog of finality settles over the scene.

All of this—regardless of the relationships between the adult children and the dying parent.

As the quote above references, science has proven that hearing is the last of the senses to go. So loved ones are encouraged to say whatever final words they want to say, even if their parent can't respond.

One can only hope that other adult children have not saved things to say that they will wish they'd said sooner in these deathbed settings. Because for a satisfying close to their parents' Act 3, adult children need to have shared their sentiments while their parents could not only respond, but understand. Even cherish and savor. The forgiveness, the affirmation, the "Me too, son."

———————

That's powerful.

The story that follows tells of Brad's poignant visit with his dying mother. It illustrates how many adult children would like to say goodbye to a beloved parent.

Brad's seventy-year-old mother lay dying of cancer. Throughout their lives, they were as close as a mother and son could be.

Her dying provided an opportunity for yet another caring conversation between two people who deeply cared for each other.

Brad agonized over how to initiate his final goodbye. Too soon, and his mom might lose her will to live. Too late, and he'd never get the chance.

He chose a Friday night to be alone with her. Nurses placed a handwritten "Do Not Disturb" sign on the closed hospital room door.

Brad had written her eulogy and held it in his trembling hands. He said, "Mom, I've written something I will share at your memorial service. I'd like to read it to you."

"That would be nice," she replied and added quietly, "I'll just lie here and close my eyes."

Several minutes and two pages later, Brad spoke the last line, then collapsed into his mom's arms. They sobbed for nearly as long as the reading took.

Then they dried their eyes and talked for an hour.

Just the two of them, looking intently at each other and saying how much they loved one another, how great their lives had been, and how they would do it all again the same way if given a chance.

They knew that not all their time together was perfect, but there was no "I wish we had done ..." or "I'm sorry I did ..."

They paused from time to time, and Brad's mom rested with her eyes closed. After one bit of prolonged silence, she opened her eyes and said weakly, "You're so nice."

She died peacefully a few days later.

If any of us are lucky, we will have an opportunity to say goodbye to our parents in much the same way Brad did.

It may be your most meaningful caring conversation.

It might well be your last.

———————————

Don't save it for the eulogy.

Start today. Prepare two lists, one that lists what you need to know and one that lists what you need to say. You'll be glad you did.

CHAPTER 6

NO ONE CAN DO EVERYTHING; **EVERYONE CAN DO SOMETHING**

"Mom had a tendency to rag on Dad and complain about him, but we girls all saw how much he did for her."

L ET'S BEGIN WITH A story about Aileen that shows how helpful it is to have a sibling orchestrate the help of family members when a crisis occurs:

Aileen e-mailed and phoned her four siblings and their spouses regularly. She provided the glue that kept them informed about their parent-related goings-on.

One day a medical crisis came out of the blue; Dad needed hospitalization and surgery. Aileen took charge, and with her guidance, the family rose to the occasion.

The gals seemed to mobilize best. They figured out what needed to be done and made sure it happened. But the guys stepped up to the plate, too.

That said, Aileen saw that some family members immediately rolled up their sleeves and asked how they could help. Others sat back and waited to be asked.

She realized she couldn't make any assumptions about who was doing what. Instead, she made sure to give explicit assignments and await confirmation that the assignments had been accepted and executed.

Dad recovered just fine, and everyone in the family felt good about their contributions to his getting back on track.

In this story, Aileen mobilizes her family to respond to a crisis, and, thankfully, all goes well. Many of your parents' growing-older needs in Act 3 won't be crisis-related, but they still must be addressed.

So how best to address them? Our old friends: anticipate, communicate, delegate, and prepare.

That's what needs to be done. But anticipate what? And delegate what?

We can help.

We've created a list of eleven of the most common needs you will most likely have. Using our personal and professional experiences, the items on this list are the main "parent-growing-older" needs your family should anticipate, discuss, and delegate to family members.

Now we don't pretend that this list is all-inclusive or definitive. But we do warrant that it is a good start.

Your personal list will reflect circumstances unique to your family. You can and should change your list whenever you see a change in need or a change in who has agreed to respond to which need.

List of 11 Most Common Needs

1. Finances
2. Healthcare decisions
3. Home maintenance
4. Errands
5. Weekly chores
6. Personal care
7. Transportation
8. First responder
9. Family communication
10. Technology
11. Research

You will be a step ahead of most families if you discuss these needs with your family and assign roles to family members before a parent-related crisis occurs.

And believe it or not, we've seen how this can turn into a fun family project that keeps everyone involved, well, involved.

Here's how it works.

Your family members become a team with a common goal of seeing that your parents have all the love and support they need. An essential step in this assignment is ensuring that each family member knows and accepts their role in achieving the goal.

How to start? Call a family meeting, electronically or in person! It's a proven way to begin the dialogue around the question, "Who can help with what?"

Get the family to start with the assumption that everyone can do something.

That said, as we saw with the "out-of-town sibling," assignments can be tricky. Often the family member who lives closest or has the best rapport with Mom or Dad gets stuck with more than his or her fair share of work.

Or maybe the lion's share of work falls on the oldest child's plate.

Your task is to make sure the assignments are distributed as evenly—and as fairly—as possible. Keep in mind that it is perfectly acceptable to ask people outside the family to fulfill individual needs.

When you complete your discussions, you might want to record your assignments in a table like the one shown here:

SAMPLE

Most Common Needs Assignments Table

Date: May 19, 2020

	Finances	Healthcare Decisions	Home Maintenance	Errands	Weekly Chores	Personal Care	Transportation	First Responder	Communications	Technologist	Researcher
Bob		√									
Mary			√	√							
Sybil									√		
Betty							√				
Gary	√										√
Sue					√						
Larry				√							
Helen								√			
Adam										√	
Jessica						√					

While you're working with your family to assign responsibilities, there is another form/list you might want to assemble: a contact list. When completed, share a copy with all who are on the list. This information fosters effective and more frequent communication among family members, and it's invaluable in times of crisis.

SAMPLE

Contact Information

Name	Relationship to Parents	Contact Information	
		Daytime phone	
		Evening phone	
		Cell phone	
		E-mail address	
		Mailing address	
		Daytime phone	
		Evening phone	
		Cell phone	
		E-mail address	
		Mailing address	

MOST COMMON NEEDS: DETAILS

Finances

"It's not that the guys didn't care; they simply didn't know what to do. They just needed direction. They felt good about helping the folks."

Money matters are relatively universal. Whether your parents are financially independent or are regularly stretching dollars to make ends meet, someone will probably have to help manage your parents' financial affairs at some point.

Many older adults view managing their money as a fierce acid test of their independence, so tread carefully. Many hurt feelings and misunderstandings can be traced directly back to discussions of parents' finances.

To help avoid such a situation, assign a family member to this need who not only has financial skills but who can also have a profoundly caring conversation about money with your parents.

The person assigned should be creative in his or her approach to minimize damage to funds...or feelings.

Money matters include asset management, tax obligations, monthly bill paying, insurance, Medicare submissions and reconciliations, pension benefits, veterans' benefits, and paperwork associated with public assistance eligibility and recertification.

The person assigned the financial responsibility should watch the weekly flow of mail to the parents' home. Wading through volumes of mail can be time-consuming, confusing, and frustrating.

Finally, realize that the financial role can end up being a full-time job.

Depending on your parents' financial circumstances and whether they have prepared a power of attorney document, you may want an attorney's services to help get things in order.

For some families, the services of a professional trust officer can also be helpful, especially if there are substantial or complicated assets, a lack of trust among family members, a reluctance on the part of your parent to relinquish control to a child, or, simply, the lack of time or talent in this area among the family members.

Hiring a professional in these areas may "pay" other benefits, too.

Consider this: if your parents have not made arrangements for someone to manage their finances and/or assets, encourage them to do so while they can make that determination rather than waiting until someone—perhaps the courts—appoints someone for them.

If your parent is hospitalized, consider asking a hospital social worker to assist. These professionals can ask this type of question (e.g., "Who manages your finances? Have you selected someone yet?") as a matter of their routine patient's finance inquiries. The hospital will have the necessary forms and access to a notary public. The hospital social worker can assist with completing any documentation.

The financial power of attorney does not need to live close to the parent. The family member assigned to manage their parents' finances might consider using one of the many auto-pay features offered by institutions for paying monthly bills. This family member might also consider setting up charge accounts as necessary and ask the business to bill them monthly. Although sometimes a sensitive subject, this is also a handy way of seeing how your parents spend their money. Our family financial manager should also be attentive to any e-mail access your parents may have to accounts and put in place any necessary controls.

One final note: keep in mind that the power of attorney authority ends the moment the parent dies. From that moment on, the person the parent has designated to be the executor of the parent's estate controls 100% of all financial matters.

HEALTHCARE DECISIONS

"Let your parent have input as to the decisions concerning their care and living arrangements. Listen to them."

Assign someone in your family to help determine your parents' healthcare wishes. Encourage your parents to designate someone as their healthcare agent while they are still able to choose. The family member designated as the healthcare agent will speak for the family when interacting with your parents' healthcare providers.

The family member designated as the healthcare agent should discuss some "what-if" scenarios and have your parents explain what they would want the family to do in various situations. Answers to these questions come through caring conversations, and they remove the guesswork from what to do at times of crisis.

Your family needs to know your parents' healthcare wishes should the occasion arise where they can't speak on their behalf. You want your parents to be in ultimate control of their destiny. This helps remove the finger of blame and the feeling of guilt.

The family member assigned this role should ask your parents questions related to each of the following:

- ○ extraordinary interventions
- ○ hospice care
- ○ life support
- ○ nursing home placement
- ○ organ donation
- ○ palliative care

The family member serving as the healthcare agent should share the parents' wishes with the rest of the family. In this way, everyone will have an idea of what will happen when the time comes.

If your parent enters a hospital without having the advance healthcare directive document in place, ask a hospital social worker to assist. If your parent is seeing an attorney about estate planning, ask the attorney to address this issue as well. Your parents will find comfort in getting their documents in order.

As with the financial power of attorney, the family member serving as their healthcare agent does not need to live close to your parents. They simply need to be available to take phone calls from healthcare providers and make the necessary decisions for your parents' care.

Home Maintenance

Issues of home maintenance will persist as long as your parents live in their own home. Sometimes sons, sons-in-law, nieces, nephews, and grandchildren will enjoy helping with these tasks.

The family members assigned to meeting this need should feel comfortable taking direction from his/her parents and managing tasks in a manner that pleases them. This last point can be a bit tricky—but it is the parents' house. So, those performing the maintenance may have to follow instructions that, well, don't make a whole lot of sense on the surface.

For example, Mom might want snow removed from her driveway before she leaves the garage. She does not wish to leave tire tracks in the snow on the driveway. Whoever is shoveling the snow must understand that it needs to be done before 9 AM, or sure as anything, Mom will be out there doing it herself.

Those assigned home maintenance tasks should live close by. Still, major home projects may involve many family members gathering from various and faraway locations to paint the house or build a new deck.

Errands

The person assisting with errands must live relatively close to the parents. Most importantly, this person needs the patience of Father Time himself. Parents sometimes insist on making several trips to a store before they deem an item—a sweater, for example—suitable for purchase. Even when they buy an article in a single trip, they can take, well, forever to do so.

Many older people like purchasing the same brand—and even the same packaging—of an item. But brands and packaging change, which may frustrate them (and sometimes the person helping them). Find a family member who enjoys shopping and can make the activity fun for the parent without talking down to them. Not everyone has these skills.

An adult child tells how his mother made a sport of running errands: "Each morning, Mother penned her to-do list and made sure by day's end that she had checked off all items on it. Managing this list kept her engaged, dynamic, and in control. Some things seemed unnecessary to me, some seemed even silly, and most were random rather than grouped for efficiency. Still, for the sake of peace-in-the-family, I decided to keep my opinions to myself."

The person assigned this task should consider catalog or online shopping as an option. Also, they should develop a list of stores that deliver. Many communities, large and small, have online ordering services and deliver groceries and sundries for a small charge.

WEEKLY CHORES

"We found that talking to each other was healthy for our family. Once we decided to be open and caring with one another, we were able to move on and focus on Dad's needs."

A time may come when your parents will need and appreciate help with everyday chores such as laundry, changing bedding, vacuuming and dusting, mowing the lawn, and preparing meals.

Family members who live close by may be assigned some of these tasks. Still, your family may also arrange for the services of a housekeeper. Finding the right one is vital. Ideally, the housekeeper will develop a lasting friendship with parents and provide frequent and fun social contact.

Meals three times a day pose a more challenging problem than housekeeping.

In some families, members take turns providing meals. They make enough meals for an entire week and put them in their parents' freezer. Then Mom and Dad can microwave the meals as needed. Also, many local restaurants deliver meals from their menus.

For families where budgets may be tight, access to regular, nutritious meals is still a priority. Almost every community has some form of congregate dining and/or home-delivered meal options.

Whoever helps with chores needs to be mindful that older persons may see others helping them as an invasion of privacy or a loss of independence. If this happens, step back, reevaluate, and proceed with caution.

Personal Care

Parents living at home may also reach a point in their lives when they need help with personal activities such as bathing, shaving, cutting their toenails, getting dressed, and going to the bathroom.

When this need escalates, especially if a parent develops incontinence, it's wise that your family begins researching in-home healthcare, assisted living, and nursing home options. Our experience proves that families should start educating themselves as soon as self-care becomes an issue so they can make informed decisions about care options and alternatives.

Ordering medication refills and setting up Mom or Dad's medications are tasks not quite as personal as the other discussed here. However, they are still essential. A family member with nursing skills who lives nearby may be best suited for this role.

Transportation

Your parent likely needs transportation to places such as the beauty shop, barber, church, grocery store, and library. This assignment can be ideal for a family member who wants to do something—but doesn't wish to take on too much responsibility. This job may be perfect for a responsible late teen driver.

Whoever is selected or volunteers must be punctual and dependable. And equally important, this person must be willing—and physically able—to help your parent in and out of the car, perhaps multiple times in one trip (see "Errands" above).

Sometimes neighbors and friends can take your parents to church. They are going anyway and may not mind stopping by for your parents.

First Responder

Any volunteer for the first responder role should be someone who lives near your parents and can be one of the first on the scene should an emergency arise. Family members, friends, or neighbors can be assigned this role.

Due to this role's "emergency" aspects, however, a family member may be the safest choice. (If this role does not go to a family member, the first responder should be told, as clearly as possible, what the various choice-of-action boundaries are. It may also not be necessary or appropriate to include this non-family person in an ongoing family medical situation.)

First responders need to determine who to contact in a crisis. They need to make reliable decisions under stress, remain calm, and buoy the spirits of others.

Communications

Keeping family informed is vital throughout your parents' Act 3. As such, find a family volunteer to take charge of family communications. He or she should begin by creating a master list of e-mail addresses, telephone numbers, and mailing addresses of family members and, as necessary, key business or other critical contacts or associates.

The communicator may relay time-sensitive or important messages and should strive to see that everyone receives the information promptly to avoid confusion.

This person need not live close to your parents.

Technologist

Many older people enjoy e-mailing and surfing the net. You should recruit a tech-savvy family member to act as a personal help desk for your parents. This way, your parents will know who to call when technical software or machinery don't work as planned.

With today's technologies, the volunteer technologist can be miles away and still access and fix your parents' computer remotely. The technologist can also help with seemingly minor adjustments that your parents might find valuable. For example, show them how to increase the size of the objects on their computer screen, demonstrate how to type letters and other correspondence in large font sizes, or even set up address lists for groups of people your parents frequently e-mail. Private family websites can be set up so family members can share news and photos.

If you need to seek computer help outside your family, try to find someone in the community that can stop by your parents' home. Tech support in person usually beats tech support over the telephone.

Researcher

Every family needs a researcher, a person with an insatiable appetite for information, who searches the Internet for information not readily available elsewhere.

This person need not be located near your parents. And this friend or family member can help the whole family make decisions by rounding up essential information on topics like possible retirement communities, assisted living centers, or nursing homes for your parents. On another tack, if your parent has been diagnosed with a disease, the researcher can help locate critical information about this condition.

There you have the most common parental situation needs in a nutshell! If it doesn't sound too self-serving, keep your copy of this book nearby, and make notations next to the various needs as they occur. You can also take comfort in knowing, through your reading and reflection, the categories of needs that will most likely arise in one form or another in your parents' Act 3. And your own!

But don't forget to get the family together and assign individuals to each common need. Use this as a chance to enhance family communication and rapport. And remember, everyone can do something!

The following story, told by a widower's son, shows us how his sister Margaret helped distribute work that had fallen on Linda's shoulders, the adult son's wife.

My dad was always partial to my wife, Linda. After Mother died, Linda and Dad became particularly close. Linda called or visited Dad daily. She planned his menus, shopped for his groceries, and kept his house clean and functioning.

As time passed, Linda became even more involved in Dad's life. She took him to medical appointments, balanced his checkbook, and waded through the monthly mailings from Medicare. As Dad's functional and cognitive abilities failed, he became more dependent on Linda, and she spent more time helping him. I appreciated what Linda was doing, but I had no idea of the extent.

When Linda and I took a week's vacation to see the kids in Ohio, my sister Margaret came from Kansas to be with Dad. When we returned, she was in a state of mild outrage.

"I'm exhausted! I had no idea! Daddy is so needy and so dependent on Linda. He's very time-consuming and, no surprise, he's demanding. I don't know how Linda has done it all this time. We need to pitch in and help."

Margaret was right. Dad's need for support, assistance, and companionship had grown significantly since Mother's death. Linda was doing it all.

As was her style, Margaret took charge and convened a family meeting via an e-mail invitation. My two brothers, their wives, and two older grandchildren were included.

Before we knew it, Margaret and Linda had charted Dad's needs to live independently. They had assigned each of us roles and tasks to play and perform in support of his needs. All the bases were covered, and no one, including the grandchildren and Steve and Ann in Alaska, left without something to do.

Margaret made the point: No one can do everything, and everyone can do something!

What if you are an only child? The insights we've shared in this chapter still apply to you and your parents. Although you don't have siblings to work with as a team to see that your parents have the support they need, there is some tongue-in-cheek good news. There won't be sibling shouting matches about parent care!

More seriously, there is also no possibility that you will be dealing with a do-nothing brother or sister. Because of this, your role can be less stressful—though not necessarily less work—than if you were in a multi-sibling family.

On a related note, in many cases, we've seen that the only adult child's spouse may take on more responsibility than he or she would have if siblings were involved. This is a situation that, in and of itself, needs careful watching.

If you have children, they can help their grandfather or grandmother in many ways, creating memorable intergenerational experiences.

Therefore, if you are an only child, it's still true that the "everyone" you enlist can do something, and keep in mind that you don't have to do it all. Don't you think this is a perfect moment to grab a pen and paper and jot down who you know who could help with what when the time comes?

CHAPTER 7

NAVIGATING THE BIG DS: DEMENTIA, DRINKING, DEPRESSION, AND DRIVING

"As Mother's dementia advanced, she actually became sweeter and more loving. What a special privilege to witness her graceful life closure."

A S WE GO THROUGH life with our parents, we are mostly unaware that they are growing older until one day in Act 3, something happens: they miss paying a bill, they leave a kettle on the burner or a burned pan in the oven, or they cause a minor fender bender.

Suddenly, we realize it: our parents might be showing real signs of aging.

Sometimes the signs mean nothing. Who hasn't, on occasion, missed a payment or forgotten a bubbling kettle when they had a lot on their mind?

At other times, though, the signs are more serious.

We refer to some of these more serious things to come as the Big Ds: dementia, drinking, depression, and driving. Let's take them one at a time.

DEMENTIA

"As sad as it is, we find the humor and keep perspective. Dad would want it that way."

We all feel we're losing it at times. We even joke we have "some-timers disease" when we forget or misplace things. Older adults are quite often super sensitive to signs they might be getting Alzheimer's (a form of dementia). One man was so bothered by the idea of Alzheimer's he invented a new condition he called "information constipation."

When family members begin to see signs, they too often fear the worst. Admittedly, dementia is frightening—but we have watched families manage it exceptionally well.

The keys to accepting or navigating this new reality involve adjusting your expectations of what your parent can or can't do—not arguing with Mom or Dad if (s)he thinks every day is Thursday. Better to go along: "Okay. It's Thursday."

And know when and where to turn for professional help.

We suggest that adult children who fear their parent is in the early stages of dementia advise their parent to see their doctor. We also recommend you gently reassure the parent by reminding them that there is a reason for hope: nearly 80% of people over 85 do not have dementia.

Does this surprise you? The fact is that the disease is often misdiagnosed.

Overmedication, dehydration, infections, and depression can all "look" like dementia in an older person. At first glance, what may appear to be an untreatable disease, even a death sentence as some see it, may be very treatable.

In short: don't guess. Knowledge is power. Fix a reassuring look on your face and get your parent to the doctor.

If your parent refuses to cooperate, do your best to determine why (s)he is reluctant, and then work with what you know. You might call your parent's doctor, explain the situation, and ask for help. The doctor could, in turn, call your parent and advise, "It's time to come in for a routine physical." If your parent won't follow your advice to seek help, ask yourself who might (s)he listen to? Have that person suggest for your parent to see their doctor.

If your parent does see a doctor—and receives a diagnosis of one form or another of dementia—stay calm. You have a framework in which to go forward.

First, begin the process of education. Be prepared for it to be harder on you than it will be on your parent.

Let's start with memory loss. Memory loss is associated with many forms of dementia—and it is a paradox. Why? Because one of the greatest sadnesses of dementia is the loss of memory. And one of the greatest blessings of this disease is the loss of memory. Look at it this way: an older person with dementia cannot process and remember all that the diagnosis will mean for them.

Now take a step back and reflect on those statements. Once you do, we believe you will come to the same (admittedly problematic) conclusion we did: This is a blessing.

It really is.

———————————

OK, with that settled, let's move on.

Next, as tempting as it might be to try to "get to the bottom" of the diagnosis, we suggest the opposite: don't spend much time on the diagnosis.

Instead, begin to accept the situation. Learn about the situation so you can live with the situation.

For example, take the longer view: things won't change dramatically overnight. You and your parent will still have many joyous times together as you navigate this journey. But be prepared to be very realistic and grounded in the fact that your parent has a disease. For example, as the following story illustrates, there will no doubt come the time when your parent will have spent a wonderful day with you—and not recall one second of it the next day.

Where is the "good side" of this situation? This: take comfort in knowing that (s)he had a wonderful time at the time, in those moments yesterday. They were happy—and happy beats unhappy hands down. They were happy yesterday. Now focus on today.

"One day at a time" as a daily compass fits this situation to a T.

Clara, Joe's wife, had Alzheimer's.

Joe, a devoted husband, dutifully took Clara for a ride in the country. Every afternoon they traveled the exact same route. Clara loved it.

Every day she rode in a brand new car, saw sights she had never seen before, and spent time with the man she dearly loved.

Joe concluded, "It didn't really matter what kind of dementia my wife had. In her reality, she had a wonderful life every single day of those last years."

Photos can help remind Mom or Dad about the memories. This then can be the basis for another meaningful day spent together—this time reminiscing.

Keep in mind that photos often remind Mom or Dad of things from their youth. And in another twist of this disease, (s)he will more easily remember events of years ago than events from the day before. But this is also a blessing: this situation can provide you an opportunity to hear more of their life stories.

Usually, people with dementia are quite content with their new reality; if so, don't fight it. Take your cues from them and try not to impose your standards because they likely won't be able to meet them.

If, for example, your mom wants to wear the same dress every day, fine. What's the problem if she is happy? Just buy eight of those dresses so there is a clean one for each day of the week—and a spare one for special occasions.

The point is this: if something needs to get done, try to accomplish it with the least disruption to your parent. And notice we said, "try." The following story illustrates how adult children's good intentions may not have the results they intend:

Jane's daughters noticed that her clothes were ragged.

Out of love for their mom, the daughters decided that while she was away for a short time, they would clean her closet and replace her ragged clothes with some nice new ones.

Their good intentions backfired. Jane was horrified when she saw "someone else's" clothes in her closet.

She complained, "Those are not my clothes. I have never worn other people's clothes, and I won't start now! Where are my clothes?"

Jane's daughters brought back their mother's ragged wardrobe.

* They might have succeeded had they replaced one old outfit at a time.

On the other hand, we won't kid you: dementia introduces situations in your family's life that you won't like, can't control, don't understand— and can't fight.

Bottom line: you and your family will need to modify outlooks, opinions, perceptions, conventions, and expectations to cope.

That said, along the way, you will have chances to be creative, as Virginia is in the following situation:

Virginia's aunt Gladys awoke in the middle of nearly every night, put on her shoes, and wandered about the neighborhood.

One evening after Gladys went to bed, Virginia hid her shoes in the closet.

Gladys would never think of going outside barefoot, so when she awoke and couldn't find her shoes, she simply went back to bed, never to wander again.

Gone are the days when adult services professionals tried to bring the cognitively impaired person back to reality with often painful truths. In the past, if a person commented that their mother had visited them the previous evening, the old method was to confront them with the harsh fact that she had been dead for several years. As might appear blindingly obvious to you, this quite often caused a great deal of sadness and anxiety for the patient, "You mean my mother died, and I missed the funeral?"

Fortunately, those days are behind us.

Healthcare professionals now realize that a patient's contentment is more important than knowing the truth, even if it means, within reason, playing along with them.

Sometimes they employ a bit of good-intentioned acting, too, as they did with Bob:

Bob was a cantankerous old guy in the nursing home.

He had many delusions, but one day he wanted to go for a swim in the community indoor pool. He would not accept the fact that he wasn't able to swim and couldn't go.

In desperation, the staff solicited help from the nursing home administrator and asked if he could take a call from Bob regarding the pool's status.

The administrator assumed the pool manager's role and simply told Bob that he was sorry. The pool was down for maintenance that day, and he wouldn't be able to swim.

Bob accepted the news. Someone had finally told him the "truth."

Sometimes families become overwhelmed with the day-to-day management of dementia. Now that you have some of the critical mile markers of living with this disease in hand, it's time to increase your education level about the condition and the next level of approaches to dealing with it.

Your parent's doctor can be an excellent resource in this regard and may, if applicable and advisable, prescribe pharmaceutical interventions for your parent. Ask the doctor to explain any possible side effects in detail.

The Alzheimer's Association is another excellent resource.

They can provide you with a wide variety of educational and informative reading material regarding the disease, its likely progression, and available and even experimental treatments.

The town or city you live in may also be a valuable resource for you. Most communities have caregiver support groups that will help you gain fresh perspectives on what other folks and groups are doing to cope and do so positively.

On another tack, this is a great time to do that family inventory we discussed a few pages back and enlist everyone's help in caring for your Mom or Dad.

For example, writing letters, sending newsy e-mails, and sharing photographs of grandchildren, nieces, and nephews can provide hours of entertainment for your parent. You will need to accept and make peace with this: Mom or Dad may read the same letter over and over and over, thinking each reading is the first. It's OK. Again, what harm is there if your parent is happy? For this reason, cards and letters are often more meaningful than phone calls.

As we wrap up this topic, it's time to share another blunt truth with you. We won't kid you; caregiving can be darn hard work. Physically, emotionally, and even spiritually.

For this reason, and to not add any concern to your parent's already complicated life, it is essential that you take care of yourself, too!

If you need a break, explore respite care for your parent with a local long-term-care or assisted-living facility. A temporary stay can help lay the groundwork for an eventual placement if care needs exceed what your family can provide.

DRINKING

"James paid Mother's bills. We became concerned when he noticed Mother's monthly liquor bill doubled."

Be honest. What role has drinking played in your family? Has alcoholism been present or prevalent? Do your parents have an occasional social drink and a nightly highball? Is there always wine with dinner? In short, what is normal for them?

Signs of their moving away from their ordinary—in the frequency or the amount of drinking—should send danger signals.

Also, always keep (politely) in mind that what Mom, Dad (or both) tell you about their drinking may not be accurate.

One way to keep a discreet eye on this is this: when you visit them, check the number of alcohol bottles or cans of beer in their refrigerator, liquor cabinet, and pantry. You don't have to measure to the exact ounce or the last can—just keep an informal eye on how much they are drinking. Red flags arise when you see your parents seeking out (or inventing) opportunities to drink.

As with any change you spot in your parent's routine, seek first to understand. If Mom's been a teetotaler her entire life and now can't seem to do without a drink or two each day, ask her politely why she's begun. You might discover she has been having a hard time sleeping at night, and the alcohol helps her nod off at bedtime. However, one thing to check would be her medications and the stipulation regarding alcohol use with them.

You also might, after a bit of research on the Internet, suggest other solutions. For example, suppose sleeplessness has become a problem for her. In that case, some light exercise during the day might help her relax and rest more soundly. Then Mom might not even feel the need for a drink.

Here's an excellent example of why it's important to seek first to understand:

Several church ladies put up a fuss when their pastor changed the time of their Sunday service.

They raised a major ruckus, but it was never clear to the pastor why they were concerned.

After some probing, he learned the ladies were upset because for years their routine had been to attend church, return to their apartments for a drink or two, and then dine at a Sunday brunch.

The Sunday service time change cut short their time for a cocktail.

They didn't have a drinking problem; they just didn't like their routine disrupted.

If alcohol has become a problem, the family will need to act as the problem is not likely to solve itself. The sooner you begin interventions, the better for everyone. Your family members' skills and comfort level—

and their personality traits and communication styles—will determine the interventions you should be willing to try.

Some parents will listen to their children's concerns and change their consumption levels. Others will deny they have a problem and will refuse to listen. In this case, you should involve their doctor, and if the problem persists, your parent may be placed in an in-patient treatment setting.

If the problem continues beyond that pale, your parent may have to be told that they can no longer live independently.

In all cases, as difficult as the situation might appear at the time, the earlier the intervention, the more positive the outcome for all.

DEPRESSION

"I wish I had known more about depression in the elderly—how to recognize it and where to get help."

One definition of depression talks about it being a response to real or imagined loss. Is it any wonder then that depression is common among older people considering the losses they experience? How would any of us feel about losing our independence, experiencing loss of control over our lives, and total or partial loss of any of our five senses, decision-making abilities, status in life, or spouse and friends? Add to that mix the side effects of medications, and we might well feel depressed.

So, what distinguishes clinical depression from a general sadness, the blues, or just being down?

Signs of depression vary from person to person. Some simply lose their interest in the world around them and are unwilling to participate in family and friends' activities. For example, Mom no longer goes to the beauty shop. Or Dad no longer meets the guys for breakfast on Wednesdays.

Perhaps your parent(s) go to bed earlier and get up later. Maybe they stay in their bedclothes for the entire day. Sometimes a parent will stop eating and experience weight loss, or sometimes they will overeat and gain weight.

Some will be unable to fall asleep or to stay asleep. Others will cry easily or become easily angered. Or perhaps your parent(s) may become confused about time and events.

In most cases, one symptom will lead to another and another.

Occasionally, a person will talk about wishing "it was over" or "ending it all." If you hear this, seek professional help. The sooner depression is named and treated, the higher the chances are for its effective management.

Many older adults are uncomfortable with the very notion of being depressed. They are from a generation that didn't address mental health issues, often believing that depression would be viewed as a weakness, a personal failing, or a defect. They might say, "I'm not depressed," or "I need to snap out of it," or "I need to toughen up."

Some adult children have success talking to their parent(s) this way: "I've noticed you seem quieter than usual and don't seem to be sleeping well. I'm wondering if perhaps we should just mention this to your doctor during our next visit?"

If you sense Mom won't be receptive to even mentioning the subject during her next doctor visit, speak privately with her doctor. Explain what you are seeing and why you feel your mom might be depressed. Let the doctor know that your mom will be reluctant to acknowledge depression. Suggest that the doctor explain the problem using the symptoms rather than the diagnosis of depression. (S)he may be able to prescribe something for your mom that will relieve the symptoms. After all, if she is clinically depressed, she is not feeling very well emotionally. Or mentally.

Here is how Hazel convinced her husband, Ralph, that an antidepressant would be good for him:

Hazel and Ralph lived in an assisted-living center. Ralph had always had a short fuse, but he became even more challenging to live with over time.

Hazel discussed the situation with the nurse and asked if she could prescribe something for Ralph that would make him less irritable. The nurse spoke to Ralph's doctor, who agreed to start him on a mild antidepressant.

When Ralph asked Hazel why he should take the pill, she said, "It helps you think better."

Without any other information, Ralph began taking the medication, and within a few weeks, he had calmed down considerably.

Hazel felt better, too.

If you know of other folks being treated successfully for depression, share this positive news with your parent. Maybe a friend who has struggled with depression is doing better with the help of medication. Perhaps your parent would value the opinion of a minister, social worker, or granddaughter.

The key takeaway here is this: don't be afraid to enlist someone's help in addressing this problem.

Your parent's doctor may have some concerns about prescribing medications for depression. As with any medication, side effects such as drowsiness or dizziness can lead to an increase in falls, and they might interfere with other medications or alcohol.

Some doctors will only prescribe something if the person agrees (s)he is depressed—and is willing to take a medication for it. The irony is that depressed people are usually the last to see that they might be depressed.

After your parent starts depression medications, remember that it will take several days or weeks to see the effects. Your parent will often say that they have stopped taking the medication after a few days because it isn't doing any good. Insist, as politely as possible, that they continue taking it. Call the doctor and have him/her firmly advise your parent to resume the medication.

Treating depression can be the best gift you and your parent will ever share. Following treatment, many older adults are once again able to enjoy their family and friends' company and participate in their previously enjoyed activities.

DRIVING

"We arranged to have the car taken away from Dad, but unbeknown to us, he ordered another one."

Asking your mom or dad to hand the car keys over to you is awkward at best, impossible at worst. Doing so puts you in a "parenting your parent" situation, as Tim discovered in the following story:

At age sixteen, freedom, power, and independence are spelled C-A-R.

Getting a driver's license and having access to a car are the rites of passage—the "Holy Grail" of adolescence.

It didn't matter how well he did on the Department of Motor Vehicles written exam or its anxiety-inducing driving test at Tim's house. Nope—at Tim's home, his dad declared him ready to drive.

Dad satisfied himself that Tim's vision, hearing, reflexes, and cognitive abilities were worthy of keys to the 1956 Buick Roadmaster Riviera.

At Tim's house, Dad gave the green light to drive and gave him a stern reminder: "Son, it would be terrible if you had an accident and hurt someone."

Fast-forward forty years, and once again, freedom, power, and independence are spelled C-A-R. And, once again, the issues are vision, hearing, reflexes, and cognitive abilities.

But now the roles are reversed. Tim now says, "Dad, it would be terrible if you had an accident and hurt someone."

Tim found himself in the difficult position of having to give the driving red light to his dad.

One morning at the coffee shop, a group of older individuals chatted about driving. A man in his early 90s recalled when he knew it was time for him to slide out from behind the wheel. "My wife and I had a cabin in northern Minnesota we loved going to every weekend in the summer. It was a straight four-hour drive there. The problem was, I couldn't drive the car straight anymore!"

We wish all older adults would voluntarily stop driving when they should. But so very often, they don't, leaving their children to agonize over when and how to convince a parent to hand over the keys.

There are strategies you can try, however. For example, a conversation that goes something like this might lead to the desired results: "Mom, how would you feel if you caused an accident that seriously hurt you or others? Do you realize how terrible this would be? And what about the stress on our family and the other driver's family? Just imagine the stress it could cause."

And there are other resources you can leverage:

○ Sometimes a friend of your parent can break the news by saying they no longer feel safe riding with him or her.

○ Some parents will listen to their doctor's advice.

○ A social worker, pastor, or another professional your parent respects as a final authority may be able to convince him or her.

You may even be able to leverage all those people and their concerns. It may help to say, "Mom, Dr. Bowman (doctor), Ann (friend and neighbor), Dick (a cousin), and Howard (the administrator) each have told you it's time you quit driving. They can't ALL be wrong, can they?"

Still, the responsibility to take the keys away from Mom or Dad will be up to you to make and to communicate. Keep this in mind: the resolve to keep one's car (and its perception of independence) can be as firm to some people as the will to live.

The staff at a retirement community told us:

> A gentleman in a retirement community took pride in the fact that stall #1 in the parking garage was reserved for his car.
>
> Though he became a bilateral amputee who uses a wheelchair in his one-bedroom apartment, he refused to sell his car and give up that stall.
>
> "By God, that's my car," he said with pride as the car keys dangled from a ring on his belt loop.
>
> The maintenance men went out quarterly and pumped air into the tires.

Some families disconnect the carburetor on their parents' car when they feel the parent shouldn't be driving. They'll say a car part is on backorder, and, eventually, the parent forgets about driving.

One delightfully demented parent, after waiting some time for the part that didn't (and wouldn't) arrive, called her favorite car dealer and said, "Bill, send over another Volvo, would you."

Another family member called the Department of Motor Vehicles (DMV) and asked that they test the father-in-law coming in that day to renew his license. He failed the parking test three times. So, the DMV politely kept his license. The father-in-law saved face—and never drove again.

Sometimes the forgetfulness associated with aging can work to a family's advantage:

Morrie was particularly resistant to giving up the keys to his car even though he had had many close calls with his driving.

He had much respect for his doctor, who told him he couldn't drive until after the twenty-fourth of the month.

For the next six months, he told his family that he would drive after the twenty-fourth.

Eventually, he forgot about driving, and the family was able to bring the car home.

Retirement centers across the country have parking lots and garages dotted with dust-caked cars that haven't been licensed or driven for years.

Many older adults know they never get back things they give up as they age. So they often hang on to what they can for as long as they can. Their reasoning is sound, as they see it: "This is just one more thing you're telling me I can't do. Well, I think I'll just keep doing it."

_____

Even if that means gazing through a window at a dust-caked car in the parking lot.

If your parent refuses to hand over the keys, it is possible to negotiate an acceptable alternative such as:

○ If you can't entirely stop your dad's driving, you might be able to convince him to reduce the frequency. Or at least ask that he stop driving after dark.

○ Some families arrange for a driver for their parents, which allows them to keep their car.

○ Van and bus services reduce the need for personal driving.

○ Taxis, cabs, Uber, and Lyft all provide viable options, as do home care agencies.

○ Some parents transition from their car to an electric golf cart.

○ Convincing parents to give or sell their car to a grandchild can also make the parent(s) feel good about giving up their vehicle. They may well be convinced that "if it's going to Billy, it will still be in the family."

The key to all three of these issues—drinking, depression, and driving—is to stop and think: "What signs am I seeing?"

You may save one or more lives—including your parent(s)'—because of what you see.

CHAPTER 8

STUFF **MATTERS**

"What a joy for Grandma to give Michael and Tammy furniture from the farm to start their first apartment. Things she loved have a new home with people she loved."

OVER A LIFETIME, EACH of us can be roughly classified by our possessions. The material items we deem valuable: jewelry, clothes, antiques, a fly rod collection, cars, paintings, sculptures, china, or a shop filled with Stanley woodworking tools.

These possessions may help reveal many of our hopes, hobbies, lifestyles, and even, in some cases, our values and beliefs. As time passes, stuff—for lack of a better term—accumulates.

Sometimes in copious dimensions.

The point is that in our daily lives, stuff matters. It has meaning and definition to us.

That said, we also know that one person's treasure can be another person's junk. An adult child tells of her mother's salt and pepper shaker collection that was precious to the mother, but perhaps not so dear to others:

My mother collected salt and pepper shakers.

It was an obsession, a passion. Whenever we traveled, or when family or friends traveled, the collection grew.

Before he died, Dad even remodeled a bedroom in their home to display her prized collection. The *Trempealeau County Gazette* once did a feature story on Mom and her nine hundred sets of shakers.

She was so proud. It was kind of cute.

When Mother died, on top of all the other things we had to do, we had to find a home for 1,800 shakers.

Not so cute.

In Act 3, adult children can't ignore the stuff in their parents' lives. Downsizing and death will each have a voice in forcing the issue.

So, think:

- ❍ What does your parents' stuff mean to them?
- ❍ What does it say about their values and how they lived?
- ❍ How will you behave toward their stuff when the time comes?

An eighty-year-old recalls: "You never forget what it felt like going to bed hungry."

We can't imagine, but we can respect the memory.

Like Cedric in the story below, many of our parents' generation grew up during the Great Depression. As children, they had very little:

Cedric was ten years old in December of 1933 when his younger brother was born.

Cedric was excited about this new addition to the family and about Christmas, just a few days away.

Times were tough on the farm during the Depression.

Cedric recalls the somber words of his father: "Son, your brother is going to be the only present you'll get for Christmas this year."

Similarly, many of our parents had very little when they first married. That West Bend waffle maker, the beat-up one with the frayed power cord that you think should be trashed, may be a symbolic possession. Its value may be as a trigger to good memories of how far your parents have come since they started their lives together.

As we grow older, memories appreciate in value.

Take some time to try to appreciate better what your parents' possessions might mean to them. At the same time, try to anticipate the potential complexity of the settlement situation—keep, sell, donate, etc.—you will inherit when dealing with this stuff after your parent(s) pass falls to you.

For example, one of the authors of this book has a mother who is a minimalist: she travels uber lightly. The author's dad, on the other hand, is a collector. He saves everything.

Every.

Single.

Blessed.

Thing.

There's an old family joke that says two pack rats got out of the business once they'd seen this father's collection of...everything.

———————

Alternatively, pack rat parents living in a double-garaged, two-story, 5,000-square-foot colonial provide their children with a different challenge than parents who have led a Spartan existence and made the downsize move to a 1,000-square-foot, one-bedroom condo on the beach already.

So let's turn back to you for a moment. Think "worst-case scenario."

○ If your parents died tomorrow, how much of their stuff would you and your siblings be left to deal with?

○ Would you have any idea what should go where?

○ Or which family member should get what?

○ Or what's of value to family and what's of worth to Goodwill?

But here is the real question. Ask yourself, "When the situation is mine to deal with, how can I honor and respect the importance of the stuff in my parents' lives and do 'the right thing' with it?"

We can learn the answer from the experience of others.

Older people can become trapped by their possessions.

Once they owned their things; now their things own them. They may have reached an age or state of health at which they should be downsizing and moving to a smaller home or a retirement community. But they can't bring themselves to part with a houseful of belongings.

They become overwhelmed and perhaps even emotional by the thought of separating from their stuff. So it becomes a barrier to moving forward.

———————

If your parents have decided to move from their home, but a year or more has gone by without them putting it on the market, that's a good sign they're having problems dealing with their stuff.

In some cases, older people can't face the thought of getting rid of their possessions because they know doing so will create conflict in their family over who gets what. So they conclude that the best way to deal with that problem is—not to deal with it. And so they remain in a home that becomes a shrine to their unwillingness to execute a decision. Even when they know it is the right one.

Even when older people do separate and relocate, the transition can carry quite an emotional impact for them and their children. The following story illustrates this point:

My mother, Ida, was born on the farm where she and my father, Alvin, spent fifty-five years of their marriage and where I grew up. A tiny lake was near the front porch of the cottage-style farmhouse.

As they grew older, Mom and Dad realized they needed to move, so they selected an apartment in town. They couldn't take all of their belongings with them, so they prepared for an auction sale with my help.

I'll never forget the farm auction. In a matter of a few hours, a lifetime of their farming possessions were sold.

I detected tears in my parents' eyes. When they sold the old hay baler, I cried too.

See, the money Dad had made from custom hay baling summers long ago had put me through college.

It's a good idea to approach your parents about dealing with their stuff while they are healthy, have the energy to do so, and can maybe even manage to have some fun in the process.

There's wisdom in the adage "You can't take it with you," so the time will come to remind your parents of that. Perhaps that will encourage your parents to give some of their treasures away at holidays, birthdays, or anniversaries. Here's how Aunt Ethel did it:

Aunt Ethel's husband was a compulsive collector and hoarder of antiques. He bought entire estates and stored them in a network of garages around town.

They had no children. When her husband passed on, Ethel was left without a pension or a 401k—just buildings full of antiques.

Ethel lived by selling piece by piece from the collection to antique dealers from across the country.

When Ethel joined her niece Pat's family for family gatherings, she brought little somethings from her collection—items carefully selected to match each member of Pat's family's interests.

Those gifts were appreciated more than anything store-bought.

And Ethel delighted in the giving.

In another situation, a grandmother chose to give away family keepsakes to each of her two children and seven grandchildren at milestone events in their lives—age eighteen and weddings, for example.

Grandma thoughtfully went through her special things, putting each in a gift-wrapped box addressed to one of us.

Included with each item was her handwritten provenance of sorts. She wrote of how she obtained the article and why it had special meaning.

She gave me her soft leather baby shoes.

Today I have the shoes, the note in her hand—and the memory of her thoughtfulness.

An excellent way to initiate a caring conversation with parents regarding their possessions can center on your family's cast of characters and their unique needs.

To start such a caring conversation, you might take this tack: "So, Mom, let's think about who in our family could use some of the things you don't use too often or at all. You know, grandson David could really use the old Ford. What would you think of selling it to him? And Mary's family just bought that cabin up north. I'm sure they could use the bedroom furniture you've stored over the garage."

Though material possessions are removed from their direct control, the parents gain a sense of control and pleasure in passing on things that are special to them. Giving to family members and friends is preferred because it is more personal than giving to a charity. That said, charities are excellent options for some stuff—and a time for using them will likely come.

And what about your mother's salt and pepper collection?

Mindful that it means more to her than anyone else in the family, you owe her a caring conversation such as: "Mom, can we talk about your salt and pepper shaker collection? It's one of a kind. How would you like us to handle it? Do you wish for us to keep it intact? Or should we divide it among the grandchildren?"

She'll be pleased you cared enough to ask—and comforted to know she has input on the eventual home(s) for her precious collection.

> "My mother told her grandchildren, 'I would welcome you letting me know which things you would like, but don't expect to get everything you want.'"

When it is time to divide possessions among family members and absent a written directive from your parents or their active presence to call the shots, your family must come to an agreement on a methodology that everyone agrees (even if somewhat reluctantly sometimes) is fair to all.

What you devise should be unique to your family. Consider what works, stick with it, keep it as positive an experience as circumstances permit, and allow enough time to do it right.

Here's an approach that didn't work well—when a sibling charged ahead without consulting others:

> Betty and her husband, Henry, had lived in the same house for forty years.
>
> They were the typical Depression-era survivors in that they were savers. Every square inch of their house had something—usually in boxes. In some rooms, things were stacked to the ceiling.
>
> Betty and Henry intended to clean things out. They would occasionally go through a box, but it took all day because they held each item and reminisced about it.
>
> Even though their children teased them about the situation and offered to come and help them clean and sort, they continued as they were.
>
> As Betty and Henry's health began to fail, their eldest daughter took charge of the situation. She started sorting, throwing, and donating much of the contents of the boxes.
>
> The remaining siblings felt cheated that they had never had the chance to see what was in those boxes.

The number of items in your parents' lifetime accumulation of stuff can be overwhelming. So it's helpful to make a list of the stuff (read: make an inventory) and then divide the stuff into three rough categories:

- ○ Stuff that has a dollar value: a coin collection, the sterling silverware, the cut glass, or first-edition books, as examples
- ○ Next, stuff that is considered family heirlooms: the blanket Grandma quilted in 1902, Grandpa's pocket watch, or the samovar that came over from Russia with the great-grandparents, as examples
- ○ Finally, stuff with high sentimental value: your baton-twirling trophy from junior high, the family photo albums, or family Bible, as examples

---

After listing the items in these categories, determine a way that is fair to everyone in your family for dividing the items. Following are some ways that families choose to do this. Realize that you don't have to use the same method for all categories. Just determine whatever works best for your family in each category of stuff.

One group of siblings decided that they would take turns selecting items. They drew numbers from a hat that determined the order in which they selected items. The oldest sibling had the honor of drawing first from the hat. They took turns choosing one item at a time until all items were spoken for.

In another situation, a couple held a garage sale when they sold their home and moved to a condominium. Everyone—family, neighbors, friends, and garage-salers—bought what they wanted at the sale, first come, first serve.

In our next story, Janice handled the dispersal of her parents' possessions with efficiency and tact:

Janice was one of eight children, and she had come to help her dad, Chet, move into an apartment.

Chet and his wife had lived in the same house for sixty years and had the usual accumulation that goes with never moving from the family home.

Janice took responsibility for cleaning out the house. She knew that her siblings would not spend much time helping her, yet she wanted to make sure they all had a part in the decision making.

She made lists of books and sent them to her siblings so they could select any that might be of interest to them.

She took digital photos of other items and sent them via e-mail so her siblings could assist in deciding the fate of their father's possessions.

For an estate with a high dollar value, some families have found it helpful to agree in advance on how much things are worth and then buy the item(s) from the estate. This works if all the family members have sufficient funds to buy what they want.

Ideally, your family should still be talking—to one another, that is—after your parents' items head to their new homes. Although everyone may not feel they got exactly what they wanted, they should feel that the process was fair. If they don't, it's essential to address that issue as soon as possible to avoid festering bad feelings.

> My grandmother asked each of us what we wanted.
>
> We told her. Privately.
>
> Then she made a list and included it with her will.
>
> Everything else was given to my mother to dispose of.

Next, here is the story of a motivated woman who devised her own inventory categories rather than use the three we suggested:

> It was no surprise to his family when Orville suddenly died at the kitchen table Good Friday evening.
>
> It was a shock, but somehow his family always knew he would never move off the farm.
>
> When Orville died, he left Myrna with nearly 50 years of rusting farm equipment and all that goes with a dairy farm operation.
>
> Myrna was overwhelmed with the suddenness of becoming a widow.
>
> There was one thing she knew: she did not want to be on that farm next winter. She took charge and started organizing the auction sale.
>
> As she sorted through sheds and garages, she took on the motto, if it's green, it's John Deere; if it's yellow, it's Minneapolis Moline; and if it's orange, it's Allis Chalmers.
>
> With her family's help, she had the auction sale ready to go less than two months after Orville's death and was settled into the house in town within six months.

We've spoken of the challenges that possessions—"stuff," as we called it—may introduce into a family setting. Still, we close by reminding you of their poignancy.

As you've seen, you need to start talking with your folks and family about who should get what, when, and how. And get it done—but keep it fun.

After one or both of your parents die, their things may well become your things, either in fact or in memory.

There's no rush to cleaning out their clothes closets or going through their photo albums, but you will likely shed a few tears when you do. Some families agree on a specific day and time to do this together, following an agreed-upon process.

There's therapy in the reminiscing the items will produce.

Savor each story; treasure each memory.

CHAPTER 9

PLACE **MATTERS**

"I moved Mother to a charming little apartment in our town. She's unhappy and blames me. What was I thinking? I guess I wasn't."

COMMONLY, OUR PARENTS LIVE in the communities where they raised their families, grew their friendships, and retired from work. They stay where things are familiar, where they feel their sense of place, their sense of belonging. They may downsize, but they stay put.

Family comes to them.

But then many older parents, often soon after retirement, pack things up and move to a region of the country that boasts year-round tee times, lots to see and do, and relatively carefree living.

Other retirees see this as a time in their lives to travel. They have spirits for adventure and discovery.

An adult child told us this story: "My parents retired, sold everything, bought a giant RV, and hit the open road to visit every national park.

I wasn't just surprised; I was stunned.

But they're having a blast, and I'll be ready for "the call" when it comes. They even have one of those bumper stickers about spending the inheritance!"

Some cultures presume that a widowed or frail parent will move in with one of their children. In today's increasingly mobile society, this happens, but less often than it used to.

> Dad was living alone and terminally ill. I brought him to live with us for his last year. The girls were gone, and it was something I could do.
>
> The circumstances were not always pleasant, but we got through it, and I think we were all made better by the experience.
>
> Dad died surrounded by people who loved him.

In today's world, options for where parents choose to live are increasingly varied. An underlying assumption here is that each partner is healthy and able to enjoy life.

So where to go?

A key consideration is this: does the location selected meet the parents' desires and needs? Kids are often surprised by their parents' choices.

But, should physical and cognitive health issues emerge, or if one partner dies, the dynamic changes, and quite often, thoughts turn to "home" where healthcare is known and "the kids are closer."

So, good adult children with the best of intentions will probably entertain these questions at some point, if only in passing:

○ Should we move Mom closer to us?
○ Should we move Mom in with us?

The answer is: it depends.

No one said this was a simple topic.

In some cases, older parents may be waiting in fear that the "moving question" will be asked of them. In other cases, they may, quite frankly, be waiting not in fear but hope.

In either case, this is a "Proceed with Extreme Caution — Homework Required!" situation.

Why?

Because moving a parent closer to you and your family, or moving a parent in with you and your family, changes your family's dynamic in ways that can be hard to foresee now. Sometimes the result is excellent. Sometimes the result is divorce.

———————————

So let's move through the next few paragraphs cautiously.

To start, candidly think through (a) the motivation(s) for the move and (b) the ramifications of the new arrangement.

- ○ Whose needs are being met?
- ○ What will it mean to all family members?
- ○ What do your parents say they need?
- ○ What do you foresee them needing?
- ○ What costs will this change trigger? You should write down the one-time and, if applicable, ongoing costs, and considered them carefully and clearly.
- ○ Are there known habits of your parent(s) that could trigger friction?

Reconcile the various perspectives, concerns, doubts, momentary enthusiasms, and answers. After the need is clear and the additional considerations have been thoroughly discussed, proceed to address the questions of how best, where best, and who best to move the topic forward.

———————————

Then begin preliminary planning for some caring conversations. But as you do so, don't forget to hold a mirror up to your life at the same time.

It is very easy for adult children to forget or to gloss over how busy their lives are. How quickly their days fill with pressing activities. How little actual downtime is available. And, to be brutally honest, the notion that "if Mother comes to live in our town, or in our house, we will have more time together" is often a faulty notion.

And as busy as most families are, there are many ways in which this situation can unravel.

- ○ Maybe Mom sees how busy you are and interprets it as the family silently rejecting her presence.

○ Or perhaps she sees how busy you are as her being an imposition.

○ Or you or some member of your family "tolerating" her presence.

○ Or you feeling "guilty" and also feeling like you had to invite her.

This situation is one where clarity of speech, honesty in expression, and a sober-eyed look at the possible upsides and downsides of an end-to-end situation must occur.

Let's presume for the moment that your parent will be relocating near you. Much has been written about the various traumas associated with relocation.

For almost any person, separating from that which is familiar, predictable, and satisfying can be a significant trauma at any age—especially in one's seventies and eighties.

Therefore, stop and think.

Is your parent the kind of person who enjoys change, is flexible, and has something of a pioneer spirit? If so, he or she might be game for a move to your community to be closer.

But you should also consider that such a person might thrive—and be even happier—in a setting with other retired people. Perhaps in a senior housing development or a planned retirement community, where others of a similar age range have moved for proximity to those of their generation and ease of access to adult children and their families.

On a related note, it's a good idea to give a trial run to a parent's idea of moving closer to adult children. This can be done around extended holiday visits, for example. It's crucial that the parent(s) experience regions of the country that are not particularly glamorous at certain times of the year: Minnesota in March or Phoenix in August.

If, on the other hand, you know your parent(s) to be timid, less inclined to take the initiative in new situations, and most comfortable with the familiar, then your loved one(s) may not be a candidate for success in a move.

Just be honest and truthful in your assessment.

Ideally, things will work out for you as they did for this adult child:

Dad and Mom prized their independence, but they wanted to be part of our lives, too.

So they moved into a retirement living center near my siblings and me.

They set up a lovely apartment. They made new friends, enjoyed the activities, joined us for church and all the kids' stuff.

Dad died knowing Mom was set with family and friends, safety and security, and all the care and service she could ever need.

He was her provider to the very end.

The older parent(s) and the well-intentioned adult child need to be brutally honest about the motivations and capacity for success. Gauging expectations is essential.

Now let's imagine how someone might react when their parent tells them they don't want to move, and the parent is vague in explaining why.

Sadly, there will be situations where a parent is not in good health and need nursing or even hospice care. You and your family need to understand that the parent simply has less ability to engage in a discussion about a move in this situation. And frankly, they are much less invested in the outcome.

Put yourself in their position. They are ill, perhaps even terminally so. It simply won't matter to them.

In this situation, it is common and appropriate to make a move that is more convenient for the adult child.

This is especially true if the older person is now a candidate for assisted living or chronic long-term nursing home care. Let's face it, a visit across town is easier for you to make than a visit across the country to manage a parent's illness and/or failing health.

Let's switch back to a brighter scenario, but one where again, you need to proceed with great caution. In this case, because things are not always what they seem.

Let's say your parent is planning on moving closer to you. There are things to think about when you shop for senior housing options in that situation. To begin with, you must learn as much as you can about any housing environment in terms of a social setting before your parent commits to moving.

For example, suppose the vast majority of the people living in the setting are native to the locale or are long-term residents and have established cliques in the social scene. In that case, your parent might have some degree of difficulty breaking in.

Result: the parent may feel socially isolated. "I don't fit in" is not a feeling you want them to have.

One way to get to know the ins and outs of a given housing situation is through a planned trial. Many retirement living communities will host your loved one for several days of a trial stay before any kind of commitment is required.

One excellent idea to ensure that a trial stay reflects all that the parent wishes the community to be is to make a list of important things to the parent. For example, suppose your parent is an avid hobbyist or an ardent bridge player. You learn that their favorite activities are not a part of the proposed community's social fabric. In that case, your loved one might be unhappy in that setting.

Let's take a step back and re-center our thinking.

There can be many advantages to the older person and adult children sharing proximity. Imagine the joy of grandchildren and grandparents who can be present at birthdays, piano recitals, confirmations, and graduations.

Consider Mary's experience:

> We brought Mary's mother, Kate, into our active household of three teenage girls.
>
> Grandma Kate had her room decorated with her things. She could quickly retreat there when the hubbub of activity in the household became too great.
>
> More often, Grandma Kate was very much a part of the girls' lives as they grew up.
>
> She's sent them all off to college and was there for their engagements, weddings, and the births of some of their children.
>
> This arrangement, unique in so many ways, was a blessing to all concerned. It was done with love, and it was done with great attention to those things that made a difference on both sides.

However, as delightful as that scene looks in our mind's eye, we need to look behind quiet nods and room temperature smiles when discussing a move with a parent. In part, this is because even little, seemingly insignificant things cause frustration, arguments, bad feelings, and result in failed experiences with the relocation of an older parent.

For example, things that are familiar and predictable are no longer there. There is a new doctor, a new local newspaper; the television and radio stations are not in sync with what they remember. The "routine things" in their lives, such as street names and where items are stocked in their grocery store, are foreign. This would be akin to you taking a job assignment in a foreign country with little preparation and a murky frame of reference.

Bad situations can also occur when the relocated adult parent becomes, by default, dependent on the adult child who invited or seduced him or her to the new environment with the promise that "we'll have so much time together."

Moves work best when older people are relocated from where they are to a setting designed for older people with program service amenities that help with the transition. These settings are good at reestablishing the parents' sense of "I am home here," and they help them become less reliant on the presence or the participation of their adult children.

Finally, leaving well enough alone might be the best response.

In other words, if you have never had a particularly close mother-daughter relationship, your mother moving nearer to you may not be the thing to do. Or if the move happens, neither party should expect the relationship to change dramatically.

If you're sensing that the road to a clear decision on this topic is fraught with doubts and second-guessing, <u>you are so right.</u>

So, the authors have chosen to close this chapter with the story of a move that worked well for an adult child, her father, and even her father's "best friend":

When my terminally ill father informed me that he was "not going anywhere" without his beloved dog, Barkley, I knew that a nursing home was out of the question.

My friends questioned my decision to move him and Barkley to my home. They were concerned that caring for my father would be too exhausting and emotionally draining.

I have to admit, I had that concern, too. However, I also did not want to spend the next few (seven) months driving the fifty miles to his home in the evenings and on weekends to help out.

Was it exhausting and emotionally draining? Yes, sometimes.

However, the times that stand out in my mind are not the difficult times. Instead, I remember when we played "Wheel of Fortune" and awarded each other a quarter when one of us was lucky enough to guess the puzzle.

Or the evenings when we shared our popcorn with Barkley and exchanged memories from years past.

And—the many visits from friends and family who gathered around my dad to share a laugh and reminisce.

Moves matter.

Look <u>very carefully</u> before you leap.

CHAPTER 10

BUILDING A **BENEVOLENT** CONSPIRACY

"I think about how much pain my mother was in for weeks without any of the five of us knowing just how bad it was (yes, she lied). I now wish that my sister and I had sat down with neighbors, friends, and relatives years ago and set up some system where we could have gotten feedback on our mother's functioning."

I T IS TRUE THAT no one can be with their parents all the time and know everything there is to know about their health and security. It's also true that, as our parents grow older, they are often less than candid, less forthright, less than complete in answering the simple question, "How are you doing?"

It seems like such a simple question. Innocent even. Harmless and genuine. But—how many times have we heard an older person say, "I don't want to be a burden," or "I don't want to bother the kids"?

———

As a result, adult children, nearby or far away, are well served to create a caring network that we call a "benevolent conspiracy."

In a traditional conspiracy, there's a person or persons that other people are out to get. The conspiracy is usually covert or clandestine.

On the other hand, in our benevolent conspiracy, people are out to help. To help you help your parents.

And the parents themselves? They are very much engaged in the conversations and decisions as anyone and are as involved as they can be and want to be.

———

Oh, and we suggest you develop your benevolent conspiracy whether or not you live in the same community as your parents. We'll show you how next.

They say a picture is worth a thousand words. So, let's draw a diagram of your benevolent conspiracy.

You diagram this conspiracy by drawing four concentric circles on a piece of paper. Write your parents' names in the innermost circle.

In the next larger circle, add the names of immediate family members. These folks are usually the first to join your conspiracy.

In the third circle, list the names of people in your parents' community who can help become your eyes and ears. This list would include your parents' neighbors, their best friends, your old friends still in town, their pastor, the mail carrier, Meals on Wheels, and the corner grocery store that delivers. All these folks can help keep an eye on your parents for you.[3]

> "Having wonderful neighbors makes life much easier for all."

You will use the fourth circle if your parents move to a care community, such as assisted living or skilled nursing. Write the names of your parents' nurses, social workers, and administrative leaders in this fourth circle.[4]

There you go: you have diagrammed your benevolent conspiracy. There's nothing more trying than long-distance worry about a loved one. With your benevolent conspiracy, you will maintain peace of mind knowing that a caring community three layers deep surrounds and supports your parents as they grow older. They will be there for your parents when you cannot.

Congratulations!

Here's when and why Greg decided it was time to form a benevolent conspiracy for his parents:

---

3 We talked about these conspiracy members in Chapter 6, "No One Can Do Everything."

4 The facility may provide some of the things you relied on family or community members to watch for, so when your parents make such a move, you can update your list of whom you're counting on for what tasks.

On a business trip, Greg, the oldest of his siblings, called his parents, who lived in a small town in Indiana.

His dad was at a Rotary meeting, but his mom was home to answer the phone. "How are you guys doing?" he asked.

His mom said, "Oh, we're just fine," but there was something about her voice that told Greg things might not be "just fine."

None of his siblings lived nearby. Greg slept fitfully that night.

The next day he called his parents' pastor and one of his dad's best friends to ask each if they would check on his folks.

Each did and reported back that things did appear "just fine." Given that assurance, Greg felt much better. Still, he realized the need to talk with his siblings and create a benevolent conspiracy for the times ahead.

Here's an essential piece of advice on this idea given to the authors: "It's important to keep the lines of communication about the parent open between caregivers and adult children."

We agreed when we were told it, and we agree 100% now.

The same thing is right about keeping communication lines open between yourself and those hand-picked members of the three outer rings of your benevolent conspiracy.

That fact leads us to this question: how do you go about narrowing down the list of people you are enlisting for your benevolent conspiracy? We knew you'd ask that, so these questions may help you form your list of candidates:

○   Who lives in town with your parents and cares about them almost as much as you do?

○   Whom do you trust?

○   Whom do your parents trust?

○   Whom do they regularly see that could spot changes in their behavior or routines should they occur?

○   Whom would you feel comfortable calling and asking to be part of this team?

Call or visit those on your list to ask them to join the conspiracy. Be as specific as you can in what you need from them, and share how they can best contact you day or night[5].

Communication among the caring community you form here and the family members you assigned to roles in Chapter 6 is essential. Everyone involved in this benevolent conspiracy should have the most up-to-date "What's Happening?" information related to your parents.

"What will our benevolent conspiracy do?" This is the first question you will be asked by all those folks you just recruited, followed quickly by "What types of things should we in the benevolent conspiracy watch for?"

Health and safety concerns are high on the list, as well as forewarnings of any of the Big Ds (dementia, drinking, depression, and driving) as we discussed in Chapter 7.

Financial scams are of growing concern. Also, more older people are using the Internet to manage their retirement portfolios through e-trading and to manage their banking. Some older people inadvertently let their insurance policies lapse. You might ask to be listed on your parents' policies and accounts as a contact to be notified if they miss a premium.

If anyone in the benevolent conspiracy sees or hears red flags in these areas, ask them to let you know.

So just how do the members of the benevolent conspiracy watch for these kinds of things?

- They might drive by your parents' house and see if the mail is getting picked up, the grass mowed, or the sidewalk shoveled.
- If they see strange cars parked in the driveway, they can investigate.
- They could call regularly just to say hi, drop by for coffee, or offer your parents rides to appointments.

Ideally, the benevolent conspiracy sends a message to your parents that says, "We care about you, and it's not a burden doing so."

---

5   As time goes by, it's nice to thank your fellow conspiracy members appropriately for what they're doing for you and your parents!

Convincing my mom to join a support group was the best thing that happened.

While family and friends were of great help to her during my dad's later years, there was something about the support group that was priceless.

Here's a situation in which a benevolent conspiracy (in this case, the staff at the assisted living center) provided guidance and counsel to the adult children:

I began to worry about Mother after a phone call in which she sounded isolated, sad, and even depressed. I had been calling regularly to check on her, and things seemed fine.

She seemed okay three months ago when she moved from home to the Fairview Assisted Living Center.

After I hung up, I called Martha, the director of nursing at Fairview, and expressed my concern. Martha quickly reassured me, "Oh, your mother's doing just fine. She's sitting in on the book study groups, coming to evening movies every Friday night, and laughing and talking with the staff and residents.

She may just be wanting a little more attention from you and your siblings."

Given that cue, my brothers and I devised a plan where one of us would stop by to visit her at least once a week.

And speaking of the care facility staff, please keep in mind that if your parent moves to a care facility, their staff is not the enemy. They have a breadth of information and experience caring for many people, so we suggest you trust them and their advice as shown in the following circumstance:

Once we accepted the reality of Dad's need for skilled care in the nursing home, we realized his caregivers were not the enemy. They were our partners in keeping our dad safe and clean and fed and loved. They were an extension of us.

We could share information, clue them in on Dad's past and his preferences with that perspective. They welcomed this and used the insights to give even better care to our dad.

To make it easier for the staff, we named our eldest sister, Sally, as the family point person. She relayed concerns between family and Dad's caregivers.

Families should appreciate the value (and the simplicity and lack of confusion) of speaking with one voice, literally and figuratively, when they have questions, suggestions, or concerns they want to share with care facility staff.

As previously mentioned, the family should designate a family member to speak for the parents. The family also needs to make a concerted effort to understand the environment in which their parents now live and how best to work within it.

So what are you waiting for? Time to start your benevolent conspiracy today! Start by making a list of who cares about your parents almost as much as you do.

And then ask them to help.

CHAPTER 11

THEN THERE WAS **ONE**

"It has been a gift getting to know a side of my father that before her death was known only by Mom."

I T'S ACT 3.

Mr. Johnson dies.

The house lights go dark.

The lights come up onto an all-new scene several months later. Mrs. Johnson is center stage.

She looks like the same Mrs. Johnson, but it's not the <u>same</u> Mrs. Johnson.

Previously shy, tentative, and retiring, *she's just auditioned for the lead in a community play.*

That can't be the mother her family knows and loves, can it? Are the rumors true that she's dating? How should her adult children react?

———

Are they shocked, stunned, embarrassed, scandalized, or supportive?

Over time, a husband and wife develop a shared identity as a couple. You know your parents only as a twosome, so upon the loss of one, you may well be meeting the other as an individual for the first time.

Most siblings have talked through, or at least thought about, the "What if Mom goes first?" and "What if Dad goes first?" scenarios. So the adult children have an idea (perhaps vague) of how Mom or Dad will react alone.

The discussion among the adult siblings goes something like this: "Dad, despite his bravado, is passive, needy, and can't match socks. If he's left alone, we will have to run an ad immediately for help for him. Mom, on the other hand, knows nothing about finances. I'll bet she doesn't even know where their checkbook is, let alone how to balance it."

Following the death of one parent, you may see a side of your surviving parent—tender, shocking, or possibly embarrassing—that you didn't expect.

"I am the new 'one,'" says the widow or widower, and the adult children begin to reform their relationships with a person they thought they knew. You may see hidden talents emerge, too, as did this adult child:

Dad seemed content to let Mom do all the cooking, so we never thought he could boil water.

It turns out he learned quite a bit from watching Mom's culinary skills during their many years of marriage, that, and all those cooking shows they watched together. Wow, can he make a delicious omelet.

This new person doesn't burst onto the "stage-of-life" immediately. Typically, there's a period of mourning and sadness that the family endures for weeks and months after the loss. But at some point in time, the surviving spouse starts to show signs of renewal. Here's the experience of an adult child who saw a "new Mom."

Dad was a great guy, but he was also a tyrant. He ruled the roost, ran the show, and wore the pants. That was clear to all of us.

Mother waited on Dad hand and foot. She even peeled his oranges. No question she loved him, but she was dependent on him to a fault. She looked to him for everything. It's just the way they did the husband-wife thing.

When Dad died, we were sure that Mother would fall apart, withdraw and fade into the woodwork. We figured we would have to take over for Dad to get her through a day.

Were we wrong!

Mother magically transformed into a modern-day woman—a social butterfly, active and independent. I suppose you could say she had suppressed those skills and abilities over the years, given Dad's dominance.

For sure, while she grieves his loss, she enjoys being her own person.

The other day she called my brother to announce she was taking a cruise. "Something Dad would never let us do!"

You go, girl.

When a parent dies, consider regrouping with your family to update the list of assignments you made in Chapter 6, "No One Can Do Everything; Everyone Can Do Something" and relook at who's part of the benevolent conspiracy you formed in Chapter 10.

I wish I had understood how much my mother motivated my father and gave him focus and purpose in life. It was strange and difficult to watch him adjust to not having her around after her death. He seemed lost and depressed.

What may become apparent soon after a parent dies is how much your parents have been covering for one another. We refer to this as "One Plus One Equals One" or complementary maladies.

For example, one parent has 20/20 vision but hears poorly, while the other is blind as a bat but can hear a pin drop a block away. Together they do fine. But when one dies, the other's difficulties may become more apparent to the family, so you may see some needs you weren't aware of.

> My parents would never go anywhere. I always thought that was my dad's influence.
>
> But now I know it was my mom.
>
> I always thought she would be willing to do anything, that he was the stick in the mud.
>
> But that wasn't the case.

You'll also be forging a new relationship with your parent. So as we discussed previously, try to seek first to understand the situation.

Then listen, communicate, and anticipate all over again. You may experience some frustrating times, but hang in there and be as understanding as you can be.

Your parent needs you more than he or she may let on as you navigate these uncharted waters for both of you.

We worry less about our parents when we have two. But as soon as one of them is gone, there's nobody at their side day after day, and things can unfold in unusual ways.

Remain encouraging.

Stay <u>positive</u>.

Love your remaining parent even more!

Do your best to understand the remaining parent's needs and desires as their life continues.

CHAPTER 12

OOPS, **TWO AGAIN!**

"They reconnected at their sixtieth high school reunion and were married two weeks later. Elder impulse? That was seven years ago!"

JUST WHEN YOU THINK things have settled down, and Dad has adjusted to the loss of your mom, things change. Dad begins seeing someone.

Your Act 3 now has a modified cast of characters that may include his lady friend and her adult children and their families.

The plot thickens!

It's healthy to express your feelings to your parent about a new relationship.

Say it.

Once.

Then, prepare to understand the meaning of the relationship as it is and on its merits.

———————————

And be supportive.

Sometimes it's easier for the adult children to accept their parents' dating if they knew their deceased parent supported or encouraged it. Here's how one woman, Jean, communicated her wishes:

Two weeks before her fiftieth wedding anniversary, Jean lay dying in the hospital of her small town. Walter, her devoted husband, refused to leave her side, so evenings he slept on a cot by her bed.

Family, visitors, and hospital staff noticed them quietly holding hands, preparing as best they could for the inevitable.

Shortly before she died, Jean began a conversation with Walter that caught him off guard.

"Walter," she said, "you've been a wonderful husband. When I'm gone, I would like you to find another woman. Don't feel you need to stay single out of respect for me."

As Walter, speechless, began to digest his wife's words, Jean drew a crumpled sheet of paper from beneath her pillow. "I'd like you to date," she said with as much of a twinkle in her eye as she could muster.

"But promise me you won't date anyone on this list!"

Following the memorial service, Walter shared the conversation with his and Jean's two children, but he never shared the list. After a year, he began dating, most assuredly none who were off limits!

"Two again" may or may not imply marriage. Still, it does assume a new, meaningful relationship that can often be as committed as marriage.

Many adult children have found that things are less complicated if their mom or dad chooses to live with their new love without getting married. This can be touchy, but you might hold back on encouraging them to rush into a marriage if you see potential problems: health, finances, or damage to family relationships, for example.

Sometimes a parent will have a firm opinion about remarriage. Women seem less inclined to want or need to remarry than men, as evidenced by the following story:

My mother is an attractive woman, always dressed well, and has a rather charming manner. I've noticed when we're out shopping or attending church, the widowers look at her with interest and flirt.

She seems to enjoy it.

"Mom, have you ever thought about marrying again?" I asked cautiously. "Because it looks like there could be suitors."

Her reply was quick, which meant to me that she had given the idea some thought.

"I'll never get married again. It would be just my luck, he would have a stroke, and I would be visiting him every day at the nursing home, just as I did with your dad, bless his soul.

"No, marriage isn't for me; at this age, it can get way too complicated. I'll stay happy going with the girls to the Friday Night Fish Fries. You know, playing the field."

That's my mom!

What if your parent begins dating someone you or your siblings don't approve of? Can you think back to your high school years when you were dating someone your parents didn't like?

Try to put yourself in your parent's shoes.

The message here is simple: celebrate it.

You might even come around to the notion that it's a wee bit selfish to think that it is a disgrace to your parents' marriage.

It is not, you know.

In the following situation, two brothers have difficulty accepting their father's dating. But Connie helps them see things in a positive light:

My parents were married for fifty-three years.

They were devoted to each other and did everything together. When Mom died, Dad didn't seem interested in anyone or anything.

He didn't smile much.

He started to look old.

Maybe he was depressed.

For sure, Dad was adrift.

When he started seeing a lady friend, my brother, Larry, and I were appalled.

Her name was Muriel, a widow. They reconnected at the funeral of a friend, I think.

Larry was distraught. I was frustrated too. Larry insisted that Dad's dating was adolescent and a public insult to Mom's memory.

Things were pretty tense.

Then Connie, Larry's wife, clued us in. "Grow up, boys! Men are wired to be connected, and your dad needs a woman in his life. You should celebrate Muriel and be happy for him. He's happy."

Larry and I had it all wrong.

Connie was right.

Dad and Muriel enjoy each other.

Dad's smiling again, and that gives us comfort. And I even think if they decide to get married...we'll be cool with it.

We tend to glamorize new relationships with, "Oh, isn't it wonderful they've found each other in their twilight years." Many new relationships work out just fine, but some don't. In this story, a daughter lost access to her mother, who found a new man in her life:

A friend of mine's mother married a man who seemed delightful at the time.

Her mother was able to travel the world and do other things she had never been able to do.

But within three years, he was a controlling tyrant and wouldn't let her do anything.

Without him.

Here's another story with the same theme:

After my father died, my mother said she would never marry again. She made my sisters and me promise that we would remind her of this should she ever even consider remarrying.

A few months later, we were in utter shock when she told us she was dating a wonderful man named Oscar.

We reminded her of what she had asked us to promise her, but she wouldn't hear any of it. She was in love, and she was going to follow her heart.

She married Oscar a few weeks later.

We met his three sons at the ceremony.

My sisters and I soon felt that we had lost our mom because she was no longer interested in our families and us.

She was too busy with Oscar.

Even our holidays had issues.

We wanted Mom and Oscar to come and spend time with our families and her grandchildren.

Instead, Mom and Oscar insisted that all of their children and grandchildren convene at their home for Christmas dinner.

Rather than providing "do" or "don't do" advice about your parent remarrying, take some time to review the following question list.

Let's "set the stage"... imagine that your mother is considering marrying a widower, Clarence, who seems in reasonably good health...

Here are some things you could talk through with your mother and siblings:

○ What happens if Clarence has a debilitating stroke and requires skilled nursing care?

  • "Mom, what would you want us to do if something happened to Clarence early in the marriage and you ended up being his caregiver? You just went through this with Dad, and now you're poised for it to happen again."

○ What role will Clarence's children play in such a situation?

  • You don't want your mom to bear the full burden of caring for him.

○ Who has medical power of attorney for Clarence?

○ Is your mother's will current?

  • What does she want to be done with her financial and material assets if she dies before Clarence?

  • Should they be divided among you and your siblings?

  • What, if anything, should Clarence receive?

○ Is Clarence's will current?

  • Ditto. Ditto.

These days, couples remarrying late in life create prenuptial agreements more often than they did in the past. These agreements address many of the questions in the previous list.

Remarriages create blended families in which new relationships will need to be established. Sometimes, the wedding may be the first time that the bride and groom's children have met. So communication lines among the children may take a while to form.

It is a fact: you never know when your single parent might form another long-lasting relationship.

Be as open, understanding, and supportive as you can.

And remember: it is your parent's life.

Not yours.

CHAPTER 13

BIGGER THAN
THE BLIZZARD

*"Little things mean so much to my parents—a call, a card,
a few flowers, or a ride in the countryside."*

SOCIAL ISOLATION AND FEELINGS of loneliness are the malnutrition of the elderly. Your parents' worlds gradually shrinks as they age. This can result in their living like survivors on a remote island. If they socialize, they may do so only with others of their generation.

This type and level of isolation mean your folks may run the risk of becoming out of touch with the world around them. They can weaken and die, especially if they perceive (rightly or wrongly) that they've been set aside from the mainstream of life and that no one cares about them any longer.

On the other hand, adult children tend to pack as many things into a day as possible. Perhaps for some people, it gives them a feeling of getting the most out of life. Older parents sometimes adopt a reverse philosophy. They seem to make the most of a day by slowing down, doing less, and sometimes even doing nothing.

An older couple was leaving church one glorious Sunday morning.

They walked slowly, holding hands, along a walkway lined with trees and flowers. They spotted some especially beautiful flowers, stopped, and leaned over to smell their blossoms.

Although this took only a few seconds, a line of church members quickly queued impatiently behind.

After a few deep breaths to inhale the fragrance, the man turned to the young couple behind him and said, "Sorry, but it took us a lifetime to learn how to do this."

During your family's Act 3, the time you spend with your parents doing even basic, simple things together can mean a great deal to them.

At the same time, the material "stuff" you give them begins to lose its impact. It just increases your parents' pile of stuff. So rather than stuff, give them your time—to them that is precious in almost any form and for any reason.

"But," you ask yourself, "time doing what?"

Let's start with something nearly everyone enjoys—ice cream[6]. You or someone else in your family could take your parents for a ride to the Dairy Queen or A&W once a week. You can't imagine how much they'll look forward to this "appointment."

They'll enjoy the ice cream cone, to be sure. But the outing isn't about the ice cream. It's about the conversations you'll have. It's about spending time together. It's about them getting out of the house and enjoying the scenery during the ride.

As the old saw relates, your actions speak louder than your words. Taking your folks out for ice cream tells them you care about them as much as you do the other things going on in your life. That's a definite win.

Andrew grew up in a small resort town that featured a bustling main street, a lakeside band shell in a shady central park, and vacation homes built along the lake's shores.

He and his family loved jumping in the car on summer evenings and going for the thirteen-mile ride around the lake.

Andrew's mom died ten years ago, but he and his dad still take the drive. His father typically won't ask to do so. Nevertheless, whenever Andrew says, "Dad, how about a ride around the lake?" he always replies, "Sure!"

It takes but half an hour to complete the ride, but in those few minutes, they relive a lifetime of memories.

Andrew dreads the day he'll take this ride alone.

But he will.

And when he does, it will bring back wonderful thoughts of his mom and dad and the time they shared driving around the lake.

---

6   The authors presume you know if your parent(s) have diabetes, and if so will make the necessary alterations in your ice cream trip. Diabetics can eat ice cream, but they need to do so safely. See the article at *https://www.healthline.com/diabetesmine/revisiting-ice-cream-and-diabetes#1* for more information.

As younger adults, it's hard for us to realize that doing something we might think of as "nothing" with our parents is actually doing something. Indeed it is.

Sitting quietly with them and listening to their stories is a tremendous gift in your parents' eyes. In their world, few things mean as much as the gift of your undivided attention. And there are plenty of ways to make that time spent together even more golden:

- ○ Take those moments to ask them questions about their childhoods, or about your childhood, too. They appreciate a chance to share meaningful memories.
- ○ Go through photo albums together.
- ○ Create a family tree and include facts and stories they remember about your ancestors.
- ○ Record these conversations with them—even transcribe the conversations. Your family will someday treasure the recordings and writings, and you will likely be surprised at the things you find out.

Walter told us, "I was amazed at the things I learned from my dad once I started asking him about the past and listening to his stories.

For example, he told me that when he dated Mom, he sometimes took her on boat rides in the hopes that this would impress her, and she'd be won over.

I was fascinated to hear him tell the story.

Never in my growing-up years did our family go on a boat ride!

Take your parent to the mall for an hour or two of shopping or attend a new store's grand opening in town. Find a bench strategically positioned for people watching and sit and observe shoppers come and go. You might be thrilled to know how this simple pleasure provides an experience for your parent to share with their friends.

A resident of a retirement community told her friends there about her trip to a new shopping mall.

"I had heard you needed to take a nap before going to save up energy for seeing all of it, and they were right. My daughter took me there last week, and I couldn't believe it."

The resident didn't buy anything, but she visited a place in town that everybody was talking about.

The trip provided something she could share at coffee. And something she could treasure for herself—time with her daughter!

You might invite your parents to a baseball game. Baseball is a relaxed-pace game that's in no hurry to end. A game can even go into extra innings, an apt metaphor for what we all long for in life.

We learned everything takes longer—so have patience.

Patience when you are going somewhere together.

Patience when you are sharing a meal.

Patience when hearing the same story—yet again.

Patience!

It's not the destination at those times. It's the journey.

The next time you're out in public, look for the family on an outing with Grandma or Grandpa, as did John in the following situation:

While my wife and I entered our favorite restaurant for an evening meal, we encountered three generations of a family readying to leave.

The grandmother looked sharp in her Burberry scarf and cashmere camel coat, her hair freshly coiffed.

She stopped to catch her breath at a booth near the door, then tottered along with a grandson at each arm.

The group inched along at her pace, respectful of her maximum speed.

All smiled and seemed to be relishing the time together while waiting for Grandma's son to bring the car to the front door.

As you watch for these moments, you'll be surprised how many you see. Experiencing and even witnessing these times of family togetherness can be quite touching and inspiring.

So to add extra enjoyment to these times with your parents, the authors offer these words of advice: prepare to be patient.

And we share a story by Linda about her mother's relaxed pace:

I'm much more like my dad than my mom in terms of motion. I like to get things done quickly.

So when I accompanied Mom shopping, I prepared myself for slowing down.

Mom looked at everything.

She picked up items, touched them, and rubbed material between her fingers. She talked to everyone in the store who would listen about the fabric, about this, and about that.

One winter day, Mom and I Christmas shopped in Minneapolis. We were strolling along a skyway when she stopped suddenly and gasped, "Oh, look at that."

She startled me. "What, Mom?"

"Look there," she replied as she pointed to a large, lighted Christmas wreath outside the walkway.

Snow was falling.

A beautiful icicle had formed in the center of the wreath, and the light was reflecting on it just so.

The scene was breathtaking, and I'm sure I would have flown right by it without notice had she not been along.

We stood for some time to marvel at the wreath.

Just the two of us.

As you do your simple things with your parents, you're sure to become frustrated now and then. That's to be expected. Take heart in these words spoken by a devoted daughter: "I may have lost my patience with Dad, but I never lost my love for him."

So, take the pledge: "I will spend more time with my parents! "

And make a date.

You'll be glad you did.

CHAPTER 14

THE SIMPLY IMPOSSIBLE PARENT

"I called Mom to tell her I loved her, and she hung up."

THE AUTHORS HAVE ENCOUNTERED two types of simply impossible parents: the one who becomes either suddenly or gradually difficult over a short period. And the one who has been difficult his or her entire life.

Let's discuss the former situation first.

If Mom has been pleasant her entire life and suddenly becomes difficult, it is time for her to see her physician. It is possible that a medical condition could be the cause.

She could be having small strokes, an infection may have set in, or she might be experiencing early signs of dementia.

One of the first symptoms families notice with dementia is that their parent becomes suspicious, blaming their family for things they can't remember. "You didn't tell me you were going to do that," or "You hid my income checks," or "I know you stole my coat."

If Mom gets a clean bill of health from her physician and remains unpleasant, you need to continue to seek to understand. Remember the adage about walking a mile in the other person's shoes:

- ○ Maybe Mom's mad at the world because she's aging, losing her independence.
- ○ Maybe she's in pain, and either doesn't want you to know it or won't take medication to treat it.
- ○ Maybe she lost a close friend through death or relocation.
- ○ Maybe someone has offended her, and she's angry at the way she was treated.

If you can't determine what's wrong, talk with the members of your benevolent conspiracy. Are they noticing the same things you are—or is Mom or Dad only angry with you?

It may be time for a caring conversation with your parent(s) to let him or her know what you are seeing and feeling and that you need his/her help to understand the situation.

Now for the parents who have been impossible their entire life.

We begin with an adult child's confession: mine. I've always been jealous of my friends who seem to have wonderful, fun, and friendly relationships with their parents. I don't, and I never have.—*Dick Edwards.*

The authors have encountered impossible parents with whom their children have had little chance of forming loving relationships.

The authors have also seen a range of parental behavior: those who blame, those who demand, those who play favorites, those who are passive-aggressive, and those who are paranoid.

○ Some parents don't want to have a thing to do with their children.

○ Some parents want their children at hand so they can manipulate them.

Relatedly, "Once a parent, always a parent," as was first introduced earlier in the book, seems to be one thing that often frustrates adult children. The authors knew a ninety-three-year-old man who scolded his son, a prominent and highly respected man in the community, for wearing shorts when he came to visit. "It's inappropriate behavior," said the father. "Men shouldn't wear shorts in public."

So let's suppose you are dealing with an impossible parent. The authors are sorry if your parent relationship isn't what you hoped—but please don't give up.

It helps to keep in mind that there are no perfect families or perfect parent-child relationships. A family that may appear idyllic to others may have unobserved levels of internal strife.

Remember: all that glitters is not gold.

Your parent may be one who some call the "Street Angel" and the "House Devil" types; in other words, parents who are saints to everyone in the world—except to their children. Here's an example:

Virginia attended a ninetieth birthday party for a longtime friend.

The friend's daughter, Lisa, flew home to attend the celebration. During the fun and festivities, Virginia said to the daughter, "Oh, Lisa, it must be great to be here with your mom. She's such a wonderful lady. My family adores her."

Lisa paused for a second, not sure what to say.

Then she replied, "You know, it's interesting to hear people talk about my mom. I don't see her that way at all.

"You and I do not know the same person."

The authors have also seen other instances where the parent isn't a devil at home, but rather isn't home at all. How many times have you heard someone describe their dad in terms similar to, "My dad was a workaholic. I never really knew him. He was always working."

For our parents' generation, the men were typically the ones making a living. At the same time, the women worked at home. Some dads became workaholics, committed every waking hour to their jobs, and therefore never developed a relationship with their children. In the following story, George tells of such a situation:

George attended a memorial service for an eighty-year-old longtime friend. A few of the deceased's colleagues shared eulogies that spoke of his greatness as a scholar, physician, and beloved man.

The stories were tender and touching; they brought tears of sorrow and laughter to many in attendance.

Following the service, George said to the man's son, "Weren't those lovely tributes to your father?"

The man looked at George, almost apologetically, and said, "Yes, they were. I wish I had known the man of which they spoke."

What can you do when you're in the middle of a situation that you feel helpless to change—such as dealing with an impossible parent?

One thing is to adjust your expectations.

If Dad has been negative his entire life, don't be surprised by his negativity as you get older.

Remember, too, that you can only do what you can do.

You and your dad likely didn't develop your current relationship overnight. Perhaps you bear some responsibility for some aspects of the relationship. Still, in most cases, it's a two-way street. As such, you might consider this tack: focus your efforts on how you can be the best adult child you know how to be—period.

Perhaps your difficult parent may be ready to let go of one or more issues that strain your relationship.

If so, are you ready for a caring conversation about them?

Be ready.

Frank's daughter Linda, one of his five children, married Nat, an African American man.

Linda and Nat lived happily together and raised two beautiful children.

Frank made it clear that Nat was not welcome in his home, and when Linda visited with her children, Frank ignored his own grandchildren.

Time passed with no signs of a change in the relationship.

Then, at age eighty-five and after fourteen years of shunning his daughter's family, Frank experienced a change of heart.

He began attending the grandchildren's sporting events.

He welcomed them and Nat to family gatherings at his home.

It took years, but he changed.

The message is: never abandon your hopes and dreams for loving family relationships.

Another good lesson to learn is this: don't let others dictate to you their definition of "a good daughter" (or a "good son").

Your mom's church circle or coffee klatch friends may say, "Well, if Mary Ann were any kind of daughter at all, she'd be up there visiting her mother every Tuesday."

That's harsh.

But, as we just discussed, these folks may have seen only your mom's "out-in-public" side. And that personality may be precisely the opposite of what you've had to contend with throughout your life. Net: her friends don't understand the entire picture. If they did, they would see why you're not there every Tuesday.

So—you don't have a great relationship with your parent(s). In that case, you might want to double-down on keeping the lines of communication open with your siblings. Just because your relationship with your parent(s) is strained, it need not be so with your siblings. Besides, they may have similar issues. On the other hand, if your parent(s) rely on them, let them know how much you appreciate what they're doing and offer to help them in any way you can.

When dealing with an impossible parent(s), be sure to let them know your priorities: your marriage, your children, your career, and your mental health.

Reinforce that as your parent(s), they are essential to you. But stress that they also need to realize that they aren't the only concern in your life.

If they make demands, be truthful in your response to those you will and won't accept. Your parents may not like your positions, but at least they will know what they are.

It's okay to hold firm.

Finances can often be a source of tension between an aging parent and their adult children, even, in some cases, when relationships are good.

But presuming your parent is impossible, you should leave the management of their finances to a third party: a trust officer, banker, personal investment manager, or attorney. This person can make monthly or quarterly statements available to ensure that finances are being adequately managed. As a bonus, this method addresses another frequent bone of contention. If your parent's giving or loaning money to family members has become a sore point, the third party can more objectively address the situation than family members.

For some adult children dealing with an impossible parent, professional counseling can provide a valuable perspective and gauge expectations.

———————————

Realistically, when Mom has been impossible for a lifetime, the only option you may have remaining is to say, "Here's my phone number," walk away, and let be what will be.

You've just put your mom in sole charge of her destiny when she's proven to be, well, impossible.

You are not abusive, and you are not neglectful.

Take comfort in knowing that you are justified in stepping aside. You are justified in doing nothing.

———————————

We realize that not all relationships end happily. And not all unfinished business gets resolved by the time your family's Act 3 ends.

After the curtain falls, however, you want to be able to say, "I honestly tried everything I could think of to better the relationship."

If you genuinely believe that, you should have no regrets after your parent(s) are gone. You may be sad for not having a relationship you had hoped for, but at least you won't feel guilty that you didn't make an effort.

Learn from this experience and apply it to your own Act 3.

CHAPTER 15

AS THE CURTAIN **FALLS**

"I know it was a big deal, but I can't honestly remember what it was.
Different things are important now."

NOW THAT YOU'VE READ this far, you should know more about helping parents grow older than the person sitting by you on the plane or standing with you at the supermarket checkout.

The authors hope the insights we've shared have not only informed and touched you but have also motivated you to proceed.

So what will you do with the time remaining in your family's Act 3? For a starter, get your family working together on a plan to support your parents through their growing-older years.

Initiate caring conversations.

Take charge and guide your family's Act 3 to a happy ending.

———————————

That said, families commonly have rifts, or fallings-out, or estrangements, even schisms. Someone did something or didn't do something, someone said something or didn't say something, and it starts.

Intense feelings of anger can fester, and good can people behave poorly. This behavior ranges from the suppressed, unspoken to the classic "Hatfields and McCoys."

The authors refer to these dynamics as "family hatchets." We strongly suggest these hatchets be buried in your private "Hatchet Cemetery" before the final scene of your parents' Act 3.

Imagine how difficult it is for the estranged sibling to rejoin the family at a time of parent crisis or at the time of dying and death. Reason enough to bury the hatchet(s).

What would be inscribed on the tombstones in your family's Hatchet Cemetery?

Here lies John's anger toward his father,
for never speaking words of affection or pride.

or

Here lies Jack's jealousy
of Tom's business success.

or

Here lies Amy's frustration with her mom
for never accepting the man she married.

The authors have heard too many sad stories of parents and children who have refused to speak and the silence that follows the parent(s) to the grave. The child lives on with regret that he or she didn't initiate an action that could have resolved the matter.

In the Judeo-Christian tradition, children are instructed to Honor your father and your mother, so that you may live long in the land the Lord your God is giving you (Exodus 20: 12, NIV). This commandment is the only one of the ten that promises something in return to those who follow it. It promises that if you honor your parents, your days will be long, and things will go well. We're not suggesting that you treat your parents lovingly solely for selfish reasons. Rather, because, as we believe you will agree, it is the right thing to do. And, you'll have fewer regrets.

While Act 3 unfolds, your children are observing how you treat your parents. After the parents die, their Act 3 ends, and a new Act 3 begins, one in which you will play the role of the aging parent.

If your children have observed you treating your parents well, they will be more likely to treat you in a way you prefer.

Each family's Act 3 ends uniquely. Like snowflakes, no two curtains fall in the same way. Though we can't always script the ending to our liking, we may have more control than we think.

An adult child tells how his family planned a fond farewell for their mother:

> Four weeks before our mother died, we didn't know it was four weeks before our mother died.
>
> Mother had just completed a round of intense chemotherapy for her cancer. My sister, Martha, believed Mother was strong enough to enjoy a weekend in Chicago. My three brothers and I agreed.
>
> Martha holds an executive position in her company. She called Mom to say, "Mom, I have a speaking engagement in Chicago. You're feeling better, why don't you come with me? I'm staying at a lovely hotel on Michigan Avenue. We'll do the weekend up right. You can get some needed rest, too. We'll even have room service."
>
> Mom said, yes.
>
> A limo met Mom and Martha at the airport and whisked them to their downtown hotel.
>
> The bellboy escorted them to their suite on the top floor. Martha could almost read Mom's thoughts: "My daughter must be important if she is treated like this."
>
> As they dressed for dinner, there was a knock at the door. "Who could that possibly be?" asked Mom.
>
> "I have no idea," said Martha. "I'm not quite ready. Can you get the door?"
>
> Mom opened the door to see me and my brothers dressed to the nines in tuxedos, beaming with smiles and extending a bouquet of roses.
>
> That weekend was all about Mom.
>
> She was the queen!
>
> We wined and dined and squired her around Chicago.
>
> We shared many memories and a few tears.
>
> It was perfect.
>
> Four weeks later, we buried our mother.

Fast forward to the day of your parent's funeral or memorial service.

How will it be?

Friends and family will be gathered. Favorite flowers and songs, and readings will be shared. Words of comfort, appreciation, and celebration will be spoken.

How will you do?

The best you can hope for is that at the close of your family's Act 3, during the service, you will experience a calm peace of mind and hear a whisper within you: "As I say goodbye, I have no regrets."

No regrets.

There's no better way for the curtain to fall on your family's Act 3.

ENCORE:
GUEST CONTRIBUTORS

Chapter 16: Who Will Take Care of Joey When We're Gone?

Mary Ann Djonne—Mary Ann Djonne—Mary Ann is mother to a special needs adult child.

Mia Corrigan—Mia is a Licensed Social Worker who has worked most of her career supporting adults with disabilities and their families.

Chapter 17: Mom, What's Happening to Grandpa?

Angie Swetland—Angie is retired Corporate Director of Customer Relations at Presbyterian Homes and Services (MN) and author of *I Know You by Heart, Navigating the Dementia Journey*, also published by Cresting Wave Publishing.

Chapter 18: And Then, Pandemic!

Jane Danner—Jane is Director of Resident Engagement and Development at Volunteers of America.

CHAPTER 16

WHO'LL **TAKE CARE OF JOEY** WHEN WE'RE GONE?

By Mary Ann Djonne and Mia Corrigan

Joey is 47 and lives with our eighty-two-year-old mother. Dad died a year ago.

Joey had a traumatic brain injury at birth and has multiple physical and cognitive limitations. He's been with Mom since the day he was born.

Joey has always lived in our family home, and our parents have supported him without any support from outside services.

Mom assists Joey with all of his daily needs and supports.

My brother and I got on with our lives and have been as supportive as Mom lets us.

She's now facing her mortality and keeps asking, "Who'll take care of Joey when I'm gone?"

How do we answer?

My sister Eleanor has Down's syndrome, is thirty-three, lives in a supported living service, and has a part-time job.

Our parents were insistent that Eleanor grow up with all the same opportunities we did. Early on, they enrolled her in every available support service and program in the community.

Eleanor loves her independence and is a fun person to be around.

Mother and Dad are getting older.

How do I get ready to assume the role of support and oversight for Eleanor as she gets older and our parents are gone?

Where to start?

As parents of adult children with disabilities face their mortality, they worry and wonder: Who'll take care of Joey when they're gone? Our job is to honor our parents by assuring them that their child with disabilities—our sibling—will be loved, provided for, included, and respected after they're gone.

Families with aging parents of an adult child with disabilities have unique questions and feelings of responsibility to "do the right thing" for their siblings and parents. They may be trying to support their parents with their changing needs, as well.

If you have a sibling with a cognitive or physical disability, then you've likely given some thought as to what will happen when Mom and Dad are gone, or as associated roles of supporting your sibling become more difficult for them to manage. As our parents age, they may not see (or be willing to admit) that it is becoming difficult to provide the same level of support they could give a few years ago.

Sometimes the other adult children need to step in to take over some things gradually. It can be tough to give up some of these roles in addition to thinking about one's mortality. We need to understand and empathize with this. It is never too early to plan and have these crucial discussions. Plan, plan, plan! Talk to your adult sibling with disabilities about their wishes, needs, and supports. Don't assume a cousin, an uncle, or a sister will step up "if something happens."

Caring conversations should include topics around needs and areas for which they may have natural supports (such as supports that Mom and Dad automatically and naturally provide in day-to-day life), as well as financial support needs, healthcare needs and wishes, living arrangements (and goals surrounding this), transportation needs, social and recreation activities (including friendships and relationships), vocational supports, and activities of daily living.

It comes down to understanding who is involved in your sibling's overall support, what resources are available and are currently in place, and their level of independence and need for help in these areas. Some agencies and tools can facilitate future planning with families.

It is critically important to consider your family dynamics. Perhaps you or one of the other siblings doesn't want to help, is unable to help, isn't comfortable having this role (just wants to be a brother or sister), or simply does not know what the supports entail.

This is OK. There is not just one path or right or wrong answer.

Take your time.

Additionally, we all may have different strengths, and this may be something to consider when planning. Perhaps one sister may do a better job of assisting with finances. At the same time, you advocate and communicate better for medical needs. Think of it this way: I go to my uncle for advice on buying a car because he is a "car guy." Knowing and recognizing each other's strengths can be a challenge for any family.

Regardless, multiple topics should be addressed when thinking about an adult child's well-being with disabilities when Mom and Dad are gone or cannot provide the same level of support they do now. Perhaps there is a sibling already extensively involved. It's essential to start a discussion together.

Consider who in your family has the most credibility with your parents and your sibling with a disability. This person may open the door to these discussions to set a solid foundation for often difficult conversations.

"Mom, Dad, sister Eleanor, we love you. We admire and respect how well you do.

"Mom and Dad, you won't be around forever, and when that time comes, we want to do the 'right thing.' We want to be prepared.

"We need you three to help us understand your wants, wishes, needs, and preferences.

"Tell us what we need to know and what we need to do, and we will."

WHERE DO I START?

At the center of these conversations is your sibling with a disability. If they are able, it is essential to center the discussion with and on them.

○ What will the death of your parents mean for them?

○ What do they want in the future?

○ What goals and wishes do they have?

○ What supports do they need?

These can be anything from formal supports and services to areas family and friends provide. These questions are essential to assess because parents often "just do things" and may not truly recognize all the help they provide today.

○ Is your sibling completely independent with things like medication management, grooming, and hygiene tasks?

○ Or do they appreciate cues and reminders with specific tasks? It is easy to make assumptions—but it is crucial to explore these kinds of details.

Some families use the services of a case manager from a public human service agency. They can assist with things such as assessing, planning, care coordination, and referral services. If your sibling has a case manager, it can help your other family members get to know them early.

Include them in planning meetings.

Ideally, you want to avoid situations where immediate needs arise, and siblings are not aware a case manager is involved. There may be other supportive services already, such as residential, in-home, or vocational services.

Develop relationships with these people now rather than when a crisis occurs. For example, if your sibling is living in a supported living service, develop a relationship with the provider, and ask to be included in planning, as your sibling wishes.

> My brother, James, has a case manager, Sarah, through the local human service agency. He has worked with Sarah for several years. My parents used to talk about Sarah, but as a young adult, I understood little about how she assisted James.
>
> After my mother passed away, my father seemed more willing to have me be involved. I now call Sarah when I have questions or concerns about James and his services.
>
> James was in full support of this and seemed to enjoy having me at his planning meetings. He has welcomed me as part of his team of supporters.
>
> I feel like perhaps my mother and father thought I was too busy with my own life and unable to be a part of his team before this, but I am glad I am more involved now.

The following sections provide an overview of important aspects of caring for an adult with special needs.

DECISION-MAKING

As you begin these kinds of discussions, it is vitally important to recognize that all adults, including individuals with disabilities, have wishes, goals, and preferences. They also have the right to make their own decisions about their healthcare, finances, relationships, where they work, where they live, and with whom.

Your sibling may or may not be able to make some of these decisions on their own.

You should look at the least restrictive method in supporting your loved ones and involve them in decisions to the extent that they can.

Involving your sibling in these crucial discussions is demonstrating your love, respect, and desire for inclusion not only to your sibling but to Mom and Dad as well.

Supported decision making (SDM) is a model that allows individuals with disabilities to retain their legal capacity and make decisions by choosing supporters to help them make choices. A person using SDM selects trusted advisors, such as friends, family members, or professionals, to serve as supporters. The supporters agree to help the person with a disability understand, consider, and communicate decisions, giving the person with a disability the tools to make informed decisions.

If SDM is not appropriate, court-appointed statuses can be used when individuals lack sufficient understanding or capacity to make or communicate informed legal or medical decisions about themselves in situations involving, for example, incapacity, guardianship, and conservatorship. Be sure to refer to the language used in your state for specific definitions and associated elements.

When in doubt, ask a lawyer.

ACTIVITIES OF DAILY LIVING

To get an idea of what your sibling has or will need support with, consider the following areas. Activities of Daily Living (ADLs) is a term used to describe actions or skills associated with basic physical needs. These skills include eating, bathing, dressing, toileting, mobility, and grooming.

Instrumental Activities of Daily Living (IADLs) are skills that require more complex planning and thinking to live independently. These skills are using the telephone, shopping, preparing meals, housekeeping, using transportation, taking medication, and managing finances.

Difficulties with ADLs and IADLs often correspond to how much help, supervision, and hands-on care and support a person needs. Some people may require only cueing, reminders, and supervision. At the same time, other individuals may need physical assistance in any or all areas. Some people do well with charts and lists; some individuals don't.

Ask yourself:

○ What tools may work or not work for your loved one?

○ What are their needs?

○ What are their preferences?

○ Are there preferred routines and schedules (e.g., they like to bathe at night and prefer showers over baths)?

It is also essential to discuss any safety concerns and areas of real or perceived vulnerability, sensory or communication needs, memory, or other cognitive impairments and needs surrounding all these topics.

We felt it essential to detail things to our son that Amelia needed support with. Although she is very independent in most of her hygiene needs, she needs some help from us due to her fine motor skills and sensory sensitivity.

I explained what this might look like: I will assist Amelia with washing her hair thoroughly at least one time per week.

I will discuss with her and assist as needed, making sure her clothes are ironed for work, help her with any buttons on her clothing, and folding down her collar.

If Amelia is open to this, she will often let me assist with brushing her teeth thoroughly once or twice per week.

Amelia may seek out this support.

At other times, I may have to ask if I can support her with this.

HOUSING

People with disabilities have choices and options for living arrangements depending upon their individual needs, budget, wishes, and wants. Perhaps your sibling is in a housing situation they are happy with, and there is no need to change their living arrangements. If they are still living with Mom and Dad, it's not too early to explore and discuss what this can look like in the future. Include your sibling when possible to discuss goals surrounding this.

Some people can live independently with minimal support from outside services. Others may live alone (or with a roommate) with more frequent outside supports to help with independent living skills such as cooking, cleaning, and budgeting. Others may live in a supported living service with 24-hour support.

Some people also receive vocational support. This can vary from intensive supports, such as a recreation-based program, to minimal support, such as assisting someone with retaining a job in the community. Some people may not need vocational help at all. If this is the case for your sibling, it's important to discuss if there will be support needed after Mom and Dad are gone, what the options are, and whom to contact.

Brian and his wife, Julie, discussed the needs of his sister, Melissa, with Mom and Dad. Melissa has a cognitive disability.

Brian and Julie live in another state 1,400 miles away. Brian said, "Julie and I have already discussed this, and we both agree that should something happen to you, Melissa will come live with us."

Mom and Dad looked at each other and said, "Melissa has a life here. She has friends, a job, and knows how to get around on the bus. This is her home. Moving her so far away might not be in her best interest."

Having addressed this assumption, they continued to discuss potential options aside from moving Melissa away from her friends and support systems.

Suppose Mom and Dad are the ones currently providing all supports to your sibling. In that case, this is a critical and potentially extremely sensitive conversation to have with them. You may need to explore and discuss other supports and services. Be careful here—this may be anxiety-provoking for Mom and Dad even to contemplate other options.

FINANCIAL

The delicate subject of personal finances invokes many questions, including:

- Who manages your sibling's finances?
- Can she manage them herself?
- If she has support, who provides it?
- What are her sources of income?
- Perhaps she receives Social Security. Does she have a representative payee for Social Security benefits?
- Does she have earned income from a job?
- Do Mom and Dad pay for some or all expenses in the family home?

Other legal steps may have been taken to handle your sibling's finances, such as a special needs trust or an ABLE account (a state-run savings program for eligible people with disabilities). These may be options you are unfamiliar with and for which you may benefit from additional learning.

Whatever the source(s) of income, discuss what level of support is needed and where there may be vulnerabilities in these areas. How does this topic look now versus possible future alternatives? Do your siblings have preferences when it comes to spending and budgeting?

Again, a lawyer (or a financial planning professional) might be of assistance when in doubt.

HEALTHCARE

The medical needs of an individual with a disability can range from mild to complex. Is there an individual selected as the authorized representative for healthcare? A firm? Does your sibling have an advance directive? If so, you may want to review their wishes, along with Mom and Dad.

Does your sibling make their own appointments and attend them independently, or does someone need to go with them to assist with things like advocating and communicating? Do they need support with the overall coordination of scheduling appointments, ordering prescriptions, keeping track of when things are due, or following up on recommendations? Ask not only your sibling but also Mom and Dad to provide you with a list of phone numbers of doctors, dentists, psychiatrists, therapists, and anyone else regularly involved with the healthcare of your sibling. It may be a bit of a bother to track this information down now—but better now than in an emergency.

SUMMARY

There are many things to think about when considering your adult sibling's ongoing needs, care, support, and wishes with a disability. By having conversations with them with a caring and compassionate attitude, you can successfully achieve the goal of telling Mom and Dad, "Don't worry... I've got this covered!"

CHAPTER 17

MOM, WHAT'S HAPPENING TO **GRANDPA?**

By Angie Swetland

NANA. GRANDMA. YAYA. PAPA. G-pa. Nonni. All are terms of affection for grandparents, names born from family tradition, or the mouths of babes as they learn to speak. The bond between grandparent and grandchild is unique. It begins with a birth and ends with a death. In between, golden memories are made.

Grandparents become the tireless playmate, indulger in chief, cookie maker, pizza chef. They are the understanding confidant, the mentor, wise counselor, co-conspirator, and the cheerleader. It does take a village to raise a child—and grandparents are the village elders.

When adult children are dealing with our aging parents' issues, our parents are, at the same time, treasured grandparents. Seeing one's beloved grandparent going from active and independent to cane, walker, wheelchair, and care setting can be frightening for all concerned.

How, then, do we prepare our children, the grandchildren, for their grandparents' aging? And for what they will see and experience as the aging process unfolds?

What are their questions?

- He's not like he used to be. What's happening?
- Will this happen to others I love? What's wrong?
- How should I act toward Grandpa? Can I hug him? Why is he drooling?
- Why doesn't Grandma remember my name? Why does she stare into space?
- What can I do to help them? To let them know that I still love them?

Difficult, no? Now pull it all together. Think about the complexity of the task being set before the children:

- ○ How to understand the many expressions
- ○ And manifestations of the aging grandparent
- ○ Observed and experienced
- ○ While trying to maintain respect, love, dignity, and the sacred grandkids-grandparents relationship
- ○ "But Grandpa is not the same!"

Yes. He has changed. But he is still your child's grandpa.

So, what are the conversations? As the parent, you are called upon to help your children understand what is happening. To help them bridge the expectations they have always had for their grandparent(s) within the limitations that age and aging have imposed upon both sets of principles—the kids and the grandparents.

As we help our children at every age face the reality of their grandparent's aging, they need four things from us: information, validation, reassurance, and encouragement.

SEEK FIRST TO UNDERSTAND

Invite your child (of any age) to express their feelings, without judgment, about what they see happening to their grandparent(s). Please do not assume you know what they're thinking. Or how they're feeling. Or what they're wondering.

Ask. And listen. What does the aging of their grandparent(s) mean to them?

Acknowledge. That you, too, have similar thoughts, feelings, and questions. Reassure them that as a family, you are in this together.

Then, ask periodically: "How do you think (Grandma's/Grandpa's) doing?"

And listen.

Somewhat counterintuitively, teenage grandchildren may need extra understanding. They are engaged in the serious business of growing up, busy searching for their voice and identity. During this time, teens need their families more than ever. While at the same time, they seek a greater and greater measure of their self-esteem from their peers. They need to fit in.

Parents and grandparents can be a source of embarrassment to their children at this stage—even when they (the parents and grandparents) fit all societal norms. The emotions teenagers must manage as a function of maturing, when combined with the feelings caused by a grandparent's decline, may be more than the child can handle.

INFORMATION AND VALIDATION

As we help children of all ages deal with aging grandparents' realities, your awareness of the child's understanding of the aging process is essential. When talking about this subject, please keep it simple.

Aging is loss. And loss is something to which everyone can relate. Over time, grandparents lose the ability to do things they used to do. They can lose the ability to remember things and life events. Often the losses of aging are not always synchronized—much less fair. Some grandparents have sharp minds and failing bodies, while others have healthy bodies and failing minds. Provide facts about your parent's current situation.

Be truthful.

But take care.

Share only as much as your child needs to hear, rather than overloading them with information. Recall that this information is loaded with possible emotional impact.

That said, children, verbally, and non-verbally are pretty good at letting parents know how much they need to know. Often, it doesn't take much to satisfy them. If Grandma's aging imposes limits on her, explain in simple terms: "Grandma's hands hurt because of arthritis, so she can't play the piano today."

REASSURANCE

Do what you can to remove or lessen your child's doubts, fears, and worries. Remind them that no one is at fault for their grandparent's condition or disease. Nor can the children "catch" what Grandma has. And yes, of course, pain and all, Grandma still loves and cherishes them.

But amid all this reassurance, beware of the time trap. When you are caring for an elder and your family, your attention is going to be divided. Whatever the age of your child, they may resent the time you devote to your parent. Not only have they lost the support they are accustomed to from their grandparent, but their time with you may be reduced as well.

Make a special effort to have some one-on-one time with your child to talk, listen, and reassure.

CONTINUED ENGAGEMENT

Encourage your child to continue to engage in meaningful ways with their grandparent. For example:

O Provide your child with ideas and tools to make each visit a success. Perhaps an old photograph album to prompt shared memories. Maybe a jigsaw puzzle, checkers, a card game, or even a craft project. Give the children that role to play.

O Have your child ask a grandparent about their childhood, young adult life, work, and family life. About life lessons learned. These conversations are relatively easy and can yield new information about your parents and their grandparents from "back in the day."

O Help your child make and bring a homemade card expressing their love for their grandparent. Or suggest they ask Grandma for a hug, keeping in mind the child's comfort level.

Remind your child that people—of all ages—need to be needed. Grandkids can help their grandparent feel needed by simply asking their opinion or advice. "Grandma, should I put raisins in my oatmeal cookies?" "I'm thinking about buying a car. Do you think I should buy new or used?"

Meredith, a high school student, and her grandma always enjoyed a close relationship. Their time together was precious.

When Grandma's physical health failed, she moved into a care setting. Her mind remained sharp.

Meredith often visited and shared news of her busy life, but she wanted to make more of their time together. Journaling became the answer. Meredith engaged her grandma in purposeful conversations to capture family history and stories that only a grandma can tell with each visit.

It was now all in writing.

Grandma was engaged; she felt needed.

Meredith's parents were amazed: "She learned things we never knew, or ever asked Mom about."

WHEN GRANDMA MOVES TO A CARE SETTING

How do you help your child and yourself if Grandma has to leave her homey, cherished space and move into a care setting with others with cognitive or physical problems?

Assisted living and nursing home communities are unfamiliar places to many. The sights and sounds can be scary for children and grandchildren. There may be long corridors, medical equipment, sometimes even unpleasant smells. When visiting, you will probably see and hear other residents with various disabilities, and this may make you and your child uncomfortable.

Though such moves are made only when necessary, families often feel sad or even guilty about them. This is when you, sandwiched between two generations, should take time to reassure yourself that each decision you have made has been with the best interests of your parent—and everyone concerned—in mind.

Then prepare your child by describing this new environment before you visit. Explain why Grandma needs the extra help this new setting provides. Plan your visit, keeping it as short or long as is comfortable for all.

WHEN GRANDPA DOESN'T REMEMBER YOUR SON'S NAME

Coping with the physical changes of aging is hard. Cognitive or mental changes can be more difficult still. When individuals develop dementia, they develop symptoms affecting memory, mood, decision-making, and communication. These changes leave everyone involved, confused, and unsure of what to expect next.

Bryce and his "Pops" have always been close. Now fourteen, Bryce is busy with friends and activities and sees his grandparents less and less.

Sure, he heard his parents talk about Grandpa's diagnosis of Alzheimer's. But he never really noticed any changes.

When the whole family got together for the Fourth of July, Bryce determined to sit down with Pops and catch up. He approached his grandpa with a wide grin, expecting the usual bear hug.

Imagine his dismay when instead, Pops exclaimed, "Bobby, have you cleaned your room?" Bryce was stunned when his grandpa called him by his dad's name.

Pops's name confusion did not stop there. He sometimes thought that his son was his brother. He called his granddaughter by his own sister's name. And he often did not recall who his daughter-in-law was at all. He knew he liked her, however. He would walk up to her and say, "Hello, you!" as he gave her a peck on the cheek.

Bryce most likely felt hurt, confused, and maybe even angry at his grandfather for his failure to remember who he was. Added to those feelings may be guilt for not staying closer to Grandpa. A teenager may struggle to name these feelings and may withdraw or act out as a result.

How do you talk to your child, whether a toddler or a teenager, about the changes that dementia brings? Let's think about this in relation to the needs we mentioned:

○ Tailor your message to the child's age. Tell a six-year-old: "Grandpa has an illness that makes him forget things sometimes. That makes me sad and hurts my feelings, too. How do you feel about it?" Some children may take the changes in stride; others will struggle. Whatever their reaction, it is essential to let the child know that you care about their feelings and that their emotions are normal.

○ Additionally, a teenager is likely to need more information than a pre-teen. The Alzheimer's Association has a list of books and videos for both young children and teens. Check out the Kids & Teens page on their website.

○ Remember that many kids have placed their grandparents on a pedestal. The idea that the mind and the insights of someone who has always been a source of wisdom are failing—can be frightening. Tell your child that diseases sometimes happen and that it is no one's fault. No one did anything wrong to make Grandpa sick. Explain that right now, no medicine can make it better. The reality is that Grandpa will start forgetting more things. All that said, the core message should be: Grandpa loves you!

○ You can use the following types of words to reassure your child: "When Grandpa sees you with your brown eyes and curly hair, he reaches into his memory and pulls out a name. That name matches how he feels about all his curly-haired boys: his brother, his son, and you, his grandson. The name may be wrong, but the feeling is right. Grandpa still loves you. His brain cannot sort through things properly anymore. But you are still in his heart."

○ Proceed with forethought. Continued engagement with their grandparent can be challenging for your child because when dementia intervenes, a grandparent may become unreliable and unpredictable.

○ Teenagers, who are desperate to belong, may be reluctant to have friends over when Grandpa is around. Or they may try to avoid Grandpa altogether. On the other hand, some teens with a hyper-responsible temperament may take on more than they can manage. They may also withdraw from school activities and even their friends to be there for you. And for Grandpa.

○ In any case, please do your best to help your child maintain a healthy balance in their interactions as they navigate this new (and often complicated) situation.

You know the importance of your parents in the lives of your children. You've watched their special relationship evolve and take on meaning over the years. Know that your child's time with their grandparents during their declining years will leave lasting impressions. Within reason and without forcing the situation, help your child make this time as positive and as loving as it can be.

CHAPTER 18

AND THEN, PANDEMIC!

By Jane Danner

C OVID-19 HAS INTRODUCED SIGNIFICANT challenges to health professionals, care facility staff, and adult children caring for older persons. Jane Danner, Director of Resident Engagement and Development at Volunteers of America—and a daughter whose mother lives in assisted living memory care—offers her professional and personal insights about navigating these uncertain times.

Finally, things were settling down, falling into place after months of difficult, sometimes contentious and agonizing, conversations with my sister, dad, and mom, to the extent Mom could engage.

Difficult decisions were made.

Mom went into dementia care fifteen miles from her town. Dad was safe at home, although struggling with daily living tasks and, profoundly, the separation from Mom after fifty-five years of marriage.

There were new routines. I called Dad daily to support and coach. My sister visited as often as she could. Dad visited Mom regularly.

The situation was not ideal, but it was manageable. We were resigned and making the best of things.

Then, the coronavirus pandemic hit.

For an adult child, living with an aging parent can be difficult. Add the reality of a pandemic, and the challenges increase.

Let's review COVID-19's implications for aging parents, their families, and professional caregivers. What are the challenges, and how can you adapt to the realities?

Whether older adults live in a private home, a congregate setting, or a care setting, COVID-19 poses possible grave effects. One of the greatest is the limited opportunities for interpersonal engagement. Social isolation and loneliness are the direct consequences of the quarantine, masking, social distancing, and lockdown required by local, state, and even federal mandates in the name of public health.

The consequences of long-term social isolation for seniors can be dangerous in the extreme: substance abuse, anxiety, depression, physical decline, mental decline, and risk for an increase in dementia. The elderly are less likely than those younger to recover from the physical, mental, emotional, and cognitive declines that they are experiencing. So many things that keep them connected, vibrant, and fit have been put on hold: attending church, taking outside classes, exercising, appointments at hair salons, and visits from family, friends, and neighbors. Additionally, there is less opportunity to be outdoors and to experience nature.

What are some options for families and care providers to help counter senior social isolation during the pandemic? What can we do when one can't go into their own mother's room, hold her hand, and talk face-to-face?

Ways in which we can meaningfully connect with an isolated loved one include:

- virtual visits and video chats
- window visits
- communications via mail/card/email
- recording and sharing videos
- arranging for pen-pals
- creating virtual events like pop-up musical presentations
- pet visits

We all want the best for the residents of any senior facility. Preserving family presence while keeping residents safe is a priority. In this regard, a key challenge is balancing residents' emotional needs and that of their families with clinical safety.

Families' choices can be daunting as they try to make the best decisions for their loved ones knowing there is risk regardless of the decision. Presuming that all concerned follow widely held protocols such as social distancing, mask-wearing, and handwashing, let's review a selected handful of commonly expressed risk/benefit concerns of professional caregivers and families alike:

- What risks does family presence pose versus the impact of family absence?
- When family visits are allowed at assisted living centers and nursing homes, who will be allowed to visit? How will visitors be selected?
- What risks are there, presuming proper protocols are observed, in taking your parent for an outside walk?
- You may decide to remove your parent from a facility to provide care in their home or yours. Are there commitments to do this by all parties involved?
- If you provide the in-home care, how long are you prepared to do so?
- If your parent lives in their home and needs in-home care, what is the risk of in-home health agency personnel exposing them to COVID-19 compared with you providing the care? This is a complicated question.

With any set of questions and considerations as intricate as those we just reviewed, there may well be unintended consequences that accompany the considerations, choices, and decisions. Make sure everyone involved understands that.

It can be challenging to weigh risks and benefits and make a decision, all while abiding by parameters set by something as uncompromising as a pandemic or the factors established by local, state, or federal health mandates.

From the other side of the situation, my peers talk to me about tremendous pressure on healthcare workers and senior-living staff. The workers continually support meaningful connections for the residents in whatever forms those connections take—and are frequently referred to as heroes. But as messengers of information on what is and is not allowed, they have a heavy burden to carry. I must emphasize that this is a responsibility they do not take lightly and one that weighs heavily on their minds, hearts, and souls.

This is a tough time. Recognize that we are in an environment where everyone—facility staff and management, you, your parent(s), are under tremendous stress. This is a pandemic whose parameters and characteristics the world has never experienced. That said, you can do things to help inform your interactions with others in the pandemic and also add substance to your conclusions and opinions:

- Ask questions. Expect complete answers.
- Read widely. Knowledge is essential.
- Demand facts. They are power.
- Seek the experience and opinions of others you respect.
- Question others' judgment if you will. But avoid questioning their motivations.
- This is a time for clear-headed thinking.

My mother lives in a memory care unit of an assisted living setting. It is sad to see her forget me and my name, something that was inevitable. Her condition saddens me, but thankfully she does not fully comprehend her situation. She will say at the end of a video chat, "Come see me when you can," neither aware of the pandemic nor that I have not been to visit her in person for months.

Though I worry about the effects of her social isolation, I am thankful for her positivity and happiness. Regardless of the progression of her dementia, she remains silly and continues to enjoy laughing. I am fortunate to have a mother whom I admire and who amazes me as she adjusts to her disease, the move from her home where she and my father lived for more than fifty years, and her transfer to an assisted living memory care.

As time passes, I see her losing the twinkle in her eye.

I try not to have regrets about the past, present, and future. Memories of times with my mother are gifts that have helped me accept the world's current state. These are unprecedented times. We are in uncharted waters doing the best we can with the knowledge we have. We have to navigate personally and professionally through issues we have never experienced. And we all need to recognize the gift of each interaction we have with our elders. Whether an adult child with an aging parent or a healthcare professional, we play many roles in dealing with our elders, pandemic or not.

Seek first to understand and then to be understood.

And go easy on yourself and others as we all try to do our best in these unprecedented times.

We're in this together!

Now, put this book down.
Call your parents and your siblings,
and start the conversations.
You'll be glad you did.

DISCUSSION GUIDE: MOM, DAD... CAN WE TALK?

Helping Our Aging Parents with the
Insight and Wisdom of Others

INTRODUCTION

Mom, Dad ...Can We Talk? lends itself to group discussion in adult learning classes, book clubs, and family gatherings where adult children can share their stories about dealing with aging parents and learn from others' experiences.

This guide is for discussion leaders. One assumption is that all participants have read the book. Another is that participants have a basic readiness to share. Some discussion areas may be more sensitive than others (e.g., questions about parents' dementia, drinking, driving, depression, et cetera) so, be cautious.

Leaders ensure that no one feels pressure to share information they would prefer not to. Be guided by the participants' comfort with the topics and their willingness to engage.

The purpose of the guide is to provide the leader with general areas for discussion based on central concepts, key perspectives, and insights presented in the book and commonly encountered concerns and circumstances confronted by adult children dealing with aging parents.

As you read the book, you may want to create your questions. You decide which questions to ask, in which sequence; and, whether to discuss one or multiple sessions.

Help each participant share their experiences and advice (what has worked for him/her; what hasn't worked) with peer adult children, and (2) learn from the other participants. At a minimum, the discussions should help them stop and think about their situation, then proceed with their evaluation, communication, navigation, and celebration.

There is no single, one-size-fits-all "best," no "right way" for adult children and aging parents. It's unique to the child, to the parent, and family.

We wish you the best in leading your discussion. Please visit our websit (*www.momdadcanwetalk.com*) and tell us know how it went.

GETTING STARTED

Seek first to understand. Ask each participant to tell a bit about their families and their aging parents. For example:

Are both parents living? How old are your parents? What are their current living arrangements? How are their health physical and cognitive health? How would they describe their current situation? How open are they to talking about their futures? Are you parents pragmatists or avoiders?

Do you have siblings? How close to your parents do you and your siblings live? Would you describe your family as closely knit or loosely knit? How many grandchildren do your parents have? Do they have close friends and neighbors? Where would you place yourself on the journey with aging parents?

CORE CONCEPTS, PERSPECTIVES, AND INSIGHTS

Perspective is how we come to view things, and insight is how we come to understand things. *Mom, Dad...Can We Talk?* offers core concepts, key perspectives, and insights to help adult children understand and manage the issues and concerns of aging parents.

Let's review a few and ask ourselves: What did I take away from these parts of the book. What spoke to me? Maybe a fresh perspective, a new insight?

- Growing Older versus Aging.
- Who does better...?
- Honor your parents...
- The Five 'ates.
- ...we want what you want.
- The need to be needed...

THE COMMONLY ENCOUNTERED

What experiences have you had, what lessons have you learned, what tips can you share on these commonly encountered concerns, challenges, and opportunities. For example,

○ Engaging and managing siblings.

○ Getting everyone, parents and siblings and care providers, "on the same page."

○ Communicating between and among those who care.

○ Dealing with the death of a parent and the survivor, dating and remarriage.

○ Navigating one of the Big Ds, like driving or dementia.

○ Organizing and monitoring care services from a geographical distance.

○ Getting parents to downsize their living space, move, or relocate to a care setting.

○ Including grandchildren in the lives of their grandparents as they age.

○ Adapting to an external reality outside your influence, like a pandemic.

○ Finding and using community-based resources, like in-home services, transportation, meals.

○ Initiating caring conversations with your parents to identify concerns and to understand their wishes.

○ Other?

WRAP-UP AND MOVE FORWARD

What were the one or two most important questions you hoped to find answers to in Mom Dad Can We Talk?

What take-home messages were there for you in Mom, Dad, Can We Talk??

Now that you've read Mom, Dad, Can We Talk? and shared in this discussion, how will you go forward differently?

What are your next steps?

Final thoughts?

Thank you for sharing.

OUR
INVITATION

Helping our parents as they grow older is a journey we can travel better together.

Please join us at *www.momdadcanwetalk.com*:

- ❍ To *comment* on the book's value to you.
- ❍ To *order* additional copies of the book.
- ❍ To *talk* with the authors.
- ❍ To *share* your experience with others.
- ❍ To *ask* your questions.
- ❍ To *receive* a book discussion leader's guide.
- ❍ To *invite* the authors to speak to your group.

We look forward to hearing from you.

DICK **EDWARDS**

D ICK EDWARDS HAS THIRTY-FIVE years of experience working closely with older adults and their families. For the last twenty years he served as administrator of Charter House, the highly acclaimed model for excellence in retirement living and long-term health care affiliated with the world-renowned Mayo Clinic in Rochester, Minnesota.

At Charter House, Dick was known for his personal interest in staff, residents, and their families, and for his accessibility as they sought his support and counsel. At Mayo Clinic, Dick conducted early research on the question, "Who does better at the business of growing older?"

Dick served in the leadership of LeadingAGE , a national organization of six thousand not-for-profit providers of older adult services. He served on the board of directors, led the organization's quality initiative, Quality First, and was in involved in the early development of the Center for Aging Services Technologies. For fourteen years, Dick served in the leadership of LeadingAGE Minnesota , a statewide association of not-for profit providers of services for older adults. His expertise and excellence in leadership in eldercare has been recognized by Mayo Clinic and LeadingAGE Minnesota, with its Lifetime Achievement Award

Dick has consulted and lectured throughout the United States and abroad on topics related to growing older and quality service to the needs of persons as they age. His professional reputation is that of a passionate visionary and an articulate, compassionate advocate for persons growing older and their families. He has traveled the country extensively speaking with over 130 audiences of appreciative adult children dealing with the issues and concerns of their aging parents.

Dick is a graduate of Luther College in Decorah, Iowa, and Case Western Reserve University, Cleveland, Ohio. He and his wife, Pat, live in West Central Wisconsin, and have three adult children and six grandchildren.

Made in the USA
Monee, IL
19 March 2021